JILL ECKERSLEY is a freelance writer with many years' experience of writing on health topics. She is a regular contributor to women's and general-interest magazines, including *Good Health*, *Bella*, *Ms London*, *Goodtimes*, *Slimming World* and other titles. *Coping with Snoring and Sleep Apnoea*, *Coping with Childhood Asthma* and *Coping with Dyspraxia*, three books written by Jill for Sheldon Press, were all published in 2003–4. She lives beside the Regent's Canal in north London with two cats.

Overcoming Common Problems Series

Selected titles
A full list of titles is available from Sheldon Press,
36 Causton Street, London SW1P 4ST, and on our website at
www.sheldonpress.co.uk

Assertiveness: Step by Step
Dr Windy Dryden and Daniel Constantinou

Body Language at Work
Mary Hartley

The Cancer Guide for Men
Helen Beare and Neil Priddy

The Candida Diet Book
Karen Brody

The Chronic Fatigue Healing Diet
Christine Craggs-Hinton

Cider Vinegar
Margaret Hills

Comfort for Depression
Janet Horwood

Confidence Works
Gladeana McMahon

Coping Successfully with Hay Fever
Dr Robert Youngson

Coping Successfully with Pain
Neville Shone

Coping Successfully with Panic Attacks
Shirley Trickett

Coping Successfully with Prostate Cancer
Dr Tom Smith

Coping Successfully with Prostate Problems
Rosy Reynolds

Coping Successfully with RSI
Maggie Black and Penny Gray

Coping Successfully with Your Hiatus Hernia
Dr Tom Smith

Coping with Alopecia
Dr Nigel Hunt and Dr Sue McHale

Coping with Anxiety and Depression
Shirley Trickett

Coping with Blushing
Dr Robert Edelmann

Coping with Bronchitis and Emphysema
Dr Tom Smith

Coping with Candida
Shirley Trickett

Coping with Childhood Asthma
Jill Eckersley

Coping with Chronic Fatigue
Trudie Chalder

Coping with Coeliac Disease
Karen Brody

Coping with Cystitis
Caroline Clayton

Coping with Depression and Elation
Dr Patrick McKeon

Coping with Down's Syndrome
Fiona Marshall

Coping with Dyspraxia
Jill Eckersley

Coping with Eczema
Dr Robert Youngson

Coping with Endometriosis
Jo Mears

Coping with Epilepsy
Fiona Marshall and
Dr Pamela Crawford

Coping with Fibroids
Mary-Claire Mason

Coping with Gallstones
Dr Joan Gomez

Coping with Gout
Christine Craggs-Hinton

Coping with a Hernia
Dr David Delvin

Coping with Incontinence
Dr Joan Gomez

Coping with Long-Term Illness
Barbara Baker

Coping with the Menopause
Janet Horwood

Coping with a Mid-life Crisis
Derek Milne

Coping with Polycystic Ovary Syndrome
Christine Craggs-Hinton

Coping with Psoriasis
Professor Ronald Marks

Overcoming Common Problems Series

Overcoming Common Problems Series

Is HRT Right for You?
Dr Anne MacGregor

Letting Go of Anxiety and Depression
Dr Windy Dryden

Lifting Depression the Balanced Way
Dr Lindsay Corrie

Living with Asthma
Dr Robert Youngson

Living with Autism
Fiona Marshall

Living with Crohn's Disease
Dr Joan Gomez

Living with Diabetes
Dr Joan Gomez

Living with Fibromyalgia
Christine Craggs-Hinton

Living with Grief
Dr Tony Lake

Living with Heart Disease
Victor Marks, Dr Monica Lewis and
Dr Gerald Lewis

Living with High Blood Pressure
Dr Tom Smith

Living with Hughes Syndrome
Triona Holden

Living with Nut Allergies
Karen Evennett

Living with Osteoarthritis
Dr Patricia Gilbert

Living with Osteoporosis
Dr Joan Gomez

Losing a Child
Linda Hurcombe

**Make Up or Break Up: Making the Most of
Your Marriage**
Mary Williams

Making Friends with Your Stepchildren
Rosemary Wells

Motor Neurone Disease – A Family Affair
Dr David Oliver

Overcoming Anger
Dr Windy Dryden

Overcoming Anxiety
Dr Windy Dryden

Overcoming Back Pain
Dr Tom Smith

Overcoming Depression
Dr Windy Dryden and Sarah Opie

Overcoming Guilt
Dr Windy Dryden

Overcoming Impotence
Mary Williams

Overcoming Jealousy
Dr Windy Dryden

Overcoming Procrastination
Dr Windy Dryden

Overcoming Shame
Dr Windy Dryden

Overcoming Your Addictions
Dr Windy Dryden and
Dr Walter Matweychuk

The Parkinson's Disease Handbook
Dr Richard Godwin-Austen

The PMS Diet Book
Karen Evennett

Rheumatoid Arthritis
Mary-Claire Mason and Dr Elaine Smith

The Self-Esteem Journal
Alison Waines

Shift Your Thinking, Change Your Life
Mo Shapiro

**Stress and Depression in Children and
Teenagers**
Vicky Maud

Stress at Work
Mary Hartley

Ten Steps to Positive Living
Dr Windy Dryden

Think Your Way to Happiness
Dr Windy Dryden and Jack Gordon

The Traveller's Good Health Guide
Ted Lankester

**Understanding Obsessions and
Compulsions**
Dr Frank Tallis

Understanding Sex and Relationships
Rosemary Stones

When Someone You Love Has Depression
Barbara Baker

Work–Life Balance
Gordon and Ronni Lamont

Your Man's Health
Fiona Marshall

Overcoming Common Problems

Coping with Childhood Allergies

Jill Eckersley

sheldon PRESS

First published in Great Britain in 2005 by
Sheldon Press
36 Causton Street
London SW1P 4ST

The author and publisher have made every effort to ensure
that the external website and email addresses included in
this book are correct and up to date at the time of going to
press. The author and publisher are not responsible for the
content, quality or continuing accessibility of the sites.

British Library Cataloguing-in-Publication Data

A catalogue record for this book is available from the British Library

ISBN 0–85969–931–5

1 3 5 7 9 10 8 6 4 2

Typeset by Deltatype Limited, Birkenhead, Merseyside
Printed in Great Britain by Ashford Colour Press

Contents

Acknowledgements

Allergy is a complex subject and I am extremely grateful to the many experts who have helped with the research for this book. Special thanks are due to the staffs of Allergy UK and Asthma UK, Margaret Cox from the National Eczema Society and David Reading from the Anaphylaxis Society. I should also like to thank Professor John Warner, Dr Jonathan Hourihane and paediatric dietitian, Carina Venter.

The real experts are the many parents I spoke to who are coping with their childrens' allergies on a day-to-day basis and who generously shared their time and expertise with me in order to benefit other parents faced with the same problems and the same choices. Without them this book would not have been written. Thank you all.

Introduction

Take a look at the notice board in any British primary school staff room and you'll almost certainly see some sort of chart showing which children, in which classes, suffer from which allergies. It's not at all unusual for two or three children in each class to have asthma and have to carry inhalers. Maybe one or more will have anaphylaxis – a life-threatening allergic reaction – and will have to keep an 'Epipen', containing adrenaline, to hand in case they are stung by a bee or wasp or come into contact with peanuts. Then there are the children with eczema, a group of diseases producing unpleasant itching, soreness, reddening and blistering of the skin. There are the hay-fever sufferers, for whom summertime and high pollen counts mean misery, or those who sneeze or wheeze if they come into contact with some kinds of flowers or the class hamster or guinea-pig. The school dinner-table can be a minefield of difficulty as teachers struggle to remember which children must not be given milk, who can't tolerate eggs, and who can't eat anything made with wheat.

What is happening to our children? Think back to your own childhood and it's unlikely that you remember quite so many allergy-related health problems. It's true that diagnosis is improving. Conditions such as asthma tended to be under-diagnosed in the past. However, it does also seem to be the case that allergic reactions are on the increase, to the point where they have even been described as an epidemic.

Some children are only mildly affected by allergies, perhaps coming out in a rash if they eat strawberries, or developing a mild wheeze if they go into a flower-shop or stroke a cat. In other, rarer cases allergies can make life very difficult, not only for the child but for his whole family. Separate meals must be prepared and special food, clothing and household products have to be bought.

The good news is that most allergic conditions can be **managed**. This book is intended to help parents, carers and all those who come into contact with allergic children to do just that. Allergy management is a partnership between doctors, nurses and other health professionals, parents, teachers and children and young people themselves. Effective treatments are available for some allergic conditions, like asthma, eczema and hay fever. In other conditions, like anaphylaxis which can be life-threatening, allergen avoidance is the main strategy.

Chapter 1 gives you the low-down on allergies generally, including as much as is known about the reasons for the rise in the incidence of these conditions. If you want to know more about **asthma**, turn to Chapter 2, which explains how this most common of childhood respiratory problems can be controlled. Chapter 3 deals with **eczema**, a spectrum of skin conditions causing dryness, itchiness, crusting, weeping and general discomfort.

Food allergy and **intolerance**, a complex and often misunderstood subject, is dealt with in Chapter 4. Chapter 5 looks at **anaphylaxis**, the life-threatening end of the allergy spectrum. In Chapter 6 we look at **hay fever**, a common but nonetheless distressing condition which blights summer and the examination season for a surprising number of young people.

Changes in our environment, from super-clean homes to an increase in the use of chemicals, are sometimes blamed for the rise in allergies. Chapter 7 has information about this controversial area. In Chapter 8 we look at the various kinds of **allergy tests** currently on offer, ranging from the standard blood and skin prick tests used by hospital clinics to tests whose value has yet to be proved. In Chapter 9, allergy experts and the major national pressure groups say what they would like to happen in the fields of allergy treatment and research in the future. Finally, Chapter 10 contains the contact details of the many organizations, from national charities to companies producing allergy-friendly products, dedicated to making life easier for children with allergies and their families.

1

What is an allergy?

If allergy cases continue to increase at the present rate, it has been claimed that as many as *half* of all Europeans will be suffering from some sort of allergy by 2015.

In the summer of 2003, the Royal College of Physicians (RCP) issued a report called *Allergy – the Unmet Need* which included the following startling statistics:

- Asthma, rhinitis (itchy, runny nose and sneezing) and eczema have increased in incidence two- or three-fold in the last twenty years.
- Anaphylaxis, the severest form of allergic reaction, which can be life-threatening, now occurs in 1 in 3,500 of the population. Hospital admissions because of anaphylaxis have doubled in the last four years.
- Food allergy is the commonest cause of anaphylaxis in children. Peanut allergy has trebled in incidence over the last four years and now affects 1 in 70 UK children. Ten years ago, this was a rare disorder.

In early 2004, a Europe-wide research project into the causes of asthma and other allergic conditions was launched, in order to co-ordinate existing research and find out once and for all why so many people – and especially children – are being diagnosed as allergy sufferers.

We don't, of course, know whether allergies *will* continue to increase at the same rate. Australian researchers recently studied a group of more than 800 primary-school children from a town 150 miles north of Sydney. Rates of allergy there had increased substantially between 1982 and 1992, as they have in Europe. Between 1992 and 2002, though, rates of asthma had actually declined while rates of other allergies like hay fever and eczema were the same. The researchers could find no reason for this apparent reduction and said it was as inexplicable as the previous increase.

Why are allergies on the increase?

This, according to allergy specialists, is the million-dollar question! There doesn't seem to be a simple answer. It is known that there are far more cases of allergy in affluent Western-type societies than there are in the Third World. Allergies may be the price we in the West pay for the way we live. Various elements of our lifestyles have been blamed, from air pollution to our well-insulated and overheated modern homes, which are breeding grounds for house-dust mites. Lack of exposure to infectious diseases in childhood, over-reliance on antibiotics, household chemicals, cigarette smoking – any and all of these have been implicated. Unfortunately, there doesn't seem to be any single theory that fits all the available facts.

Take the problem of air pollution. Is the air in British cities really more polluted today than it was fifty years ago when the great London smog of 1952 killed over 4,000 people?

Or is the rise in allergies something to do with the *type* of air pollution, with sulphur dioxide, carbon monoxide, nitrogen dioxide and ozone from traffic fumes replacing the smoke from coal fires and factory chimneys? Researchers found that when East and West Germany were re-unified in 1989, the levels of allergies and asthma in polluted East German cities had actually been lower than they were in the West. In recent years, the East Germans have caught up. In Britain, teenage asthma is more common in country areas than it is in towns, and levels of pollutants like ozone and nitrogen dioxide (NO_2) vary from place to place for no apparent reason. According to British Society for Allergy and Clinical Immunology figures, Manchester had levels of ozone and NO_2 at 30 and 93 respectively, which were roughly twice those of central London, at 16 and 56. A tiny village near Beachy Head in Sussex recorded higher levels of ozone, at 64, and the remote Strathvaich Forest in north-east Scotland has even higher ozone levels at 72. Glasgow's ozone levels, at 34, seem relatively respectable, even though the city has the UK's highest levels of NO_2, at a scary 120.

Our centrally heated and well-insulated modern homes are ideal breeding grounds for house-dust mites, a common cause of childhood allergy. The fact that today's children are more likely to stay in and play computer games than play out on busy streets has led to a belief that indoor living is to blame. However, it's worth remembering that in Australia and New Zealand, countries known

2

for their generally healthy outdoor lifestyles, allergy levels are even higher than they are in Britain.

Another suggested reason for the rise in allergies is something called the 'Idling Immune System' theory, which suggests that children's immune systems, now that they no longer have to fight the infectious diseases so common in the past, are producing more of the TH-2 white cells which cause allergy problems. Third World countries, where infectious diseases are still widespread, have lower rates of allergy.

Could excessive hygiene be to blame? It is known that children who grow up on farms suffer from fewer allergies, possibly because they are exposed to farmyard dirt and animal dander from an early age. The so-called 'Hygiene Hypothesis', suggested by an epidemiologist called David Strachan in 1989, suggests that children in 'too-clean' homes, and especially those not exposed to germs brought home by older brothers and sisters, are more likely to develop allergies. Recently, however, experts in infectious diseases have begun to fight back against this idea, pointing out that there's no acceptable level of 'safe' dirt in the home and that a relaxation in standards of cleanliness could lead to more infections like food poisoning.

Other theories have linked the rise in allergies to increased use of paracetamol to treat childhood fevers, lack of the mineral selenium in the diet, even the rise in obesity. It is known that babies of mothers who smoke are more likely to have breathing difficulties, including asthma. Research on all these possible causes, and on the effect of diet in pregnancy, is still going on.

Even Prince Charles has expressed concern, claiming in a newspaper article in February 2004 that we have become allergic to the Western way of life and that overeating, lack of exercise, our obsession with hygiene and exposure to thousands of untested chemicals are 'conspiring to weaken our defences against the environment'.

How serious are allergies?

Most allergic conditions are not life-threatening and can be treated, allowing the sufferer to lead a normal or near-normal life. However, they can be unpleasant, frightening and distressing. Even something like hay fever can make children's lives a misery and can be particularly difficult for teenagers to cope with, as the hay-fever season tends to coincide with exam time!

Other allergies *are* actually life-threatening. People do die of asthma attacks and the charity The Anaphylaxis Campaign was set up by a concerned parent who lost his young daughter to an undiagnosed peanut allergy.

Living with a seriously allergic child is not easy, as Melanie has discovered. Her 5-year-old son Dylan has severe eczema and asthma. He is also allergic to cats and dogs, house-dust mites, grass pollen and many household chemicals.

'We haven't had more than two hours' sleep at a time since he was born,' she admits.

His hands are very badly affected with cracked and bleeding skin. This affects him at school as he has trouble holding a pen and he can't play with sand, water or play-dough like the other children. He has problems socially too. The other kids don't want to hold his hands, and if he goes out to tea, or to a party, I have to ring and ask if there are animals in the house. Just being in a home where there is a cat or dog makes his face swell up and his eyes close.

I have mild asthma myself and am allergic to cats and dogs. If I touch them, my eyes start to itch and my skin goes blotchy – but Dylan suffers far more. His dad has hay fever too. I took all the dietary advice about avoiding peanuts and so on when I was pregnant, and breast-fed Dylan for six months, but it didn't seem to make any difference. It never crossed my mind that he would be so badly affected.

What is a true allergy?

One difficulty is that the word 'allergy' is often used in its popular sense – to refer to any kind of unpleasant reaction to a food or substance. A true allergic reaction, however, is one which involves the body's **immune system**.

An allergy is an inappropriate response by the immune system to a substance which, in non-allergic people, is harmless.

The substance concerned could be grass pollen, egg white, a prescribed drug such as penicillin, or even cat or dog hair. The human immune system is designed to react in this way to genuine 'attackers' like viruses and bacteria. However, if your child has inherited, or developed, a tendency to become allergic (this tendency is known as **atopy** and may run in families, though it does not always do so) her immune system reacts the same way when she comes into contact with particular **allergens**, such as the substances listed above. To make it all more complicated, an individual's immune system doesn't always respond in exactly the same way to the same allergen, or with the same degree of severity.

When a susceptible child comes into contact with allergens, his immune system produces a large amount of the **allergy antibody**, **Immunoglobulin E** or **IgE**. This results in the kind of symptoms we call an 'allergic reaction' – reddening and inflammation of the skin, a streaming nose, narrowed airways which make breathing difficult, and tissue swelling. In the case of a **food allergy** (see Chapter 4) the reaction usually happens quickly – either immediately the offending food is eaten or within about 30 minutes.

The presence of the IgE antibodies is characteristic of a true allergic response and can be checked out with a 'skin prick test' or a blood test. No antibodies mean that, strictly speaking, there is no allergy. If your child suffers from a bad reaction – sickness, stomach pains, a skin irritation – and proves not to be allergic, then the problem may be better described as **intolerance**, or even **sensitivity**.

What is an intolerance?

Intolerance is a reaction which does not involve the immune system, and where the symptoms may appear much later, up to six days later in some cases. Much less is known about the mechanisms involved in food intolerance, and the usual tests for allergies don't show the presence of IgE antibodies. Usually the best way to diagnose food intolerance is by an 'elimination diet' – removing the food you suspect of causing the problem for a week or two and then re-introducing it in small quantities to see if the effect is the same. Elimination diets are often complex to follow and should always be supervised by a qualified paediatric dietician.

Other forms of intolerance are caused by an individual's inability to digest a particular substance. One of the commonest is lactose, the natural sugar found in milk and milk products. It's estimated that about one in ten British people don't produce enough of the enzyme lactase, which digests lactose, so that they suffer from stomach pain and diarrhoea if they drink a lot of milk. However, the immune system is not involved in this reaction and many lactose-intolerant people can drink some milk without ill-effects.

Some children are also sensitive to compounds in particular foods – the caffeine in coffee might make them jumpy, for example. Parents of 'hyperactive' children sometimes find that excluding additives, most notably tartrazine (labelled E102), from their child's diet helps to calm them down. (For more about hyperactive children and diet, see Chapter 4.)

Can allergies be cured?

At the moment there is no cure for allergic conditions. The aim of most treatments is to help sufferers to **manage** their condition so that they can live a normal life. Allergy management is often a combination of drug or other treatments – for instance, asthmatic children carry inhalers which are very successful in controlling the worst symptoms – and lifestyle changes. Some of these are no more than common sense and are not too difficult to achieve. Pure cotton clothing, anti-allergy bedlinen and non-toxic paints and household cleaning products are widely available. If your child is allergic to cats or dogs, keeping pets is out, though you may have more problems if your child is so severely allergic that he reacts to sitting next to a cat-owning child in school. It is also becoming much easier to feed an allergic child a balanced diet, as substitutes for the most common allergens, like wheat and dairy products, are increasingly easy to find in supermarkets as well as health-food shops.

Do children grow out of allergies?

It is very hard to predict whether an individual child will grow out of a particular allergy. Asthma is more common in children than adults. Most available research suggests that children less seriously affected tend to 'grow out of it', while those with severe asthma tend not to, but there are always exceptions. Eczema is extremely common in babies and young children, affecting about one in five British schoolchildren. However, about three-quarters of these grow out of their eczema around the time of puberty, for reasons which are still unclear. Hay fever, by contrast, is rarely a problem for very small children but affects about a quarter of all teenagers. Older people do seem to suffer from fewer allergies. In other words, most allergic conditions are unpredictable, and this can cause problems in itself, as 16-year-old Kerry explains.

I've had eczema since I was 3. I can remember being smothered in oils and creams when I was little and having to wear gloves so that I wouldn't scratch my skin. In primary school I had patches of very flaky skin but it does seem to have got better as I've got older.

The trouble is, I can never tell when I am going to have a flare-up. I can be all right for months and then suddenly I'll have a bad reaction. It happened when I went to my cousin's wedding. I don't know if it's caused by stress or worry.

I also have mild asthma, and have to use an inhaler. We have a cat and a dog at home and I find if the cat sits on my lap for too long my chest starts to feel tight. I get hay fever too and have to carry tablets and a big packet of tissues in my school bag. Luckily my teachers are pretty understanding, and so are my friends.

I sometimes wish I didn't have it but mostly I don't think about it, I just get on with my life.

It's quite common for children to have more than one allergy – eczema and asthma, hay fever and possibly one or more food allergies. All are caused by the same basic mechanism, the body's immune system reacting to substances it perceives as harmful.

'We still don't know why a child develops a *particular* allergy,' says Dr Jonathan Hourihane, who is a paediatric allergist and Assistant Director at the Wellcome Trust Clinical Research facility in Southampton.

It tends to depend which allergens he is exposed to. We have problems in Britain with house-dust mites which they don't have in Arizona. British children develop allergies to peanuts, milk or fish while Japanese children develop allergies to buckwheat or rice. In either case, the allergic response is the same.

Dr Hourihane sees young patients with all kinds of allergies, some local, some from further afield, and can offer advice on allergen avoidance as well as the best medication for rhinitis or asthma control. He feels that face-to-face advice from a specialist is helpful as it's tailored to the individual, and he also sounds a note of caution.

I spend quite a lot of time de-constructing unnecessary diets for young patients. With the best of intentions, parents often exclude foods from their child's diet without evidence that this is helpful. For example, I have seen children with peanut allergies with peas also excluded from their diets, or children who can't tolerate dairy products not eating eggs either. It's vital that parents take proper advice from a dietician. Children only get one chance to grow and need a proper balanced diet.

Allergy treatments

The fact that there is no cure for most allergies doesn't mean that they can't be treated. Sometimes medication is available and can make a tremendous difference. Preventer and reliever inhalers are generally very good at controlling asthma (see Chapter 2).

Emollient creams and lotions and topical steroids are effective treatments for eczema (see Chapter 3). Anti-histamines can help in treating hay fever (see Chapter 6).

In other cases, allergen avoidance and lifestyle changes can be the best way of managing allergic conditions. Obviously, some allergens are easier to avoid than others. Pollen and house-dust mites are everywhere; animal dander (the mixture of hair and saliva which leads to an allergic response in many sensitive children) is rather easier to avoid. Wheat and dairy products are common allergens and more difficult for your child to avoid than, say, strawberries, tomatoes or shellfish.

Anti-IgE treatment and immunotherapy

Immunotherapy, sometimes known as 'desensitization', is a treatment which is widely used outside Britain against some kinds of allergies, for instance bee and wasp stings. It works by injecting a small amount of protein derived from the particular allergen into the patient, increasing his tolerance. In the 1980s this kind of treatment was used in Britain but proved fatal in a few cases. Dr Jonathan Hourihane and his team are currently involved in safety trials and are hoping to re-introduce immunotherapy as a safe and reliable treatment for some kinds of allergy.

'It is available all over the world apart from Britain. We have moved on from the problems which existed in the 1980s,' he says. 'In Europe, oral immunotherapy is also being used so no injections are necessary and that should also be suitable for treating children. In the next two or three years it may be available in Britain too.'

Complementary medicine

Allergy experts are always cautious when considering complementary treatments, pointing out that most have not been through the rigorous clinical trials that pharmaceutical products need to undergo before they are approved for use. If you are considering treating your allergic child with complementary therapies, it's important to consult a reputable practitioner – for instance, one who is a member of the National Institute of Medical Herbalists or the Acupuncture Council (contact details on pp. 94–5). Organizations like Asthma UK and the National Eczema Society can also give advice on complementary treatments, some of which have been found to benefit some children. **Always tell your GP and allergy specialist that you are thinking of trying complementary therapies. No reputable therapist should suggest you abandon conventional medication in favour of an unproven 'alternative'.**

2
Asthma

Asthma is the leading cause of the hospitalization of children all over the world and is also the main reason why children have to miss school. According to Asthma UK (formerly the National Asthma Campaign), as many as 1.4 *million* children in Britain are being treated for asthma at any one time. It is about three times as common as any other childhood condition.

The UK has the highest number of teenage asthma cases in Europe – more than twice as many as France and Germany – and the third highest in the world after Australia and New Zealand. The reasons for this are still unclear.

What is asthma?

Asthma is a condition in which an allergic response causes the airways to become swollen, inflamed and sore. In addition they produce more mucus. The combination of swelling and mucus makes the airways narrower, so it becomes increasingly difficult for enough air to flow into the lungs, causing the characteristic 'wheeze'. Coughing and shortness of breath can also be symptoms of asthma.

To make diagnosis more complicated, though, not all 'wheezy' breathing in children is caused by classic allergic asthma. Nor do all asthmatic children wheeze – the symptoms vary from child to child, and may also be different at different times in the same child. Professor Martin Partridge, Chief Medical Adviser to Asthma UK, points out that for this reason it can be quite difficult to diagnose asthma in very young children. Frequent episodes of coughing, wheezing and breathlessness can be caused by other conditions: for example,

- virus infections;
- bronchiolitis, another viral disorder where the bronchioles, narrow air passages in the lungs, become ultra-sensitive and filled with mucus;

- croup – which also tends to produce a characteristic 'barking' cough.

Causes of asthma

Like all other allergic conditions, the incidence of childhood asthma has increased a great deal over the last thirty years. The Global Allergy and Asthma European Network, launched in February 2004, is to be the co-ordinating body for all the many hundreds of research projects aimed at finding out exactly why.

As already explained in Chapter 1, many children with asthma come from so-called **atopic** families – those with a tendency to develop allergic conditions ranging from asthma and eczema to hay fever or food allergy. There is a hereditary element involved but the link is not clear-cut. Asthma is one of several 'complex inheritable conditions', like diabetes and high blood pressure, in which a number of genes rather than just one contribute to a child's susceptibility. Scientists are still trying to discover precisely which genes are responsible for the tendency to develop asthma.

In Chapter 1, we looked at the various elements which *may* be implicated in the recent rise in the incidence of asthma and other allergic conditions. These range from air pollution, both outdoor and indoor, to the so-called 'Hygiene Hypothesis' which states that our centrally heated, well-insulated, super-clean modern homes may be partly to blame. It is possible that several of these factors need to be present and combine to produce a case of asthma in a child from an atopic family. At the moment there doesn't seem to be any one-size-fits-all explanation, as Professor Partridge points out.

If an individual is predisposed to developing asthma, it may need only a minor environmental trigger to bring on the disease.

In an individual who has only a minor susceptibility, there may need to be a significant number of triggers before the condition develops.

Can asthma be prevented?

If you know you and/or your partner have a tendency to asthma or another allergic condition, there are steps you can take which may help to avoid passing on the condition to your children. These include:

- Minimize your exposure to allergens like house-dust mite and pet dander while you are pregnant.
- Avoid peanuts and peanut products during your pregnancy or while you are breast-feeding your baby. Mums-to-be should eat a healthy, balanced diet containing items from all the major food groups. For the latest advice on healthy eating in pregnancy, call the Sainsbury's/WellBeing Helpline (contact details on p. 88).
- Give up smoking, if possible before you even become pregnant. Experts in the respiratory health of babies and children all agree that this is one step that would absolutely guarantee better lung health. Research shows that the longer mums-to-be continue to smoke, the more likely it is that their babies will suffer from breathlessness and wheezing during the first six months of their lives. The BMA report *Smoking and Reproductive Life*, published in early 2004, estimated that between 14,000 and 19,000 babies are born underweight in Britain each year. Low-birthweight and premature babies are particularly prone to health problems, including respiratory difficulties.
- Continue to breast-feed your baby for at least four months. Some asthmatic mothers worry that their asthma medication could affect their babies but expert opinion is that the minute quantities present in breast milk are unlikely to be harmful.
- Minimize your baby's exposure to cold germs in the first six months if you can.

If your child has asthma

Although an asthma attack can be frightening, the good news is that today's range of treatments are extremely effective. The aim of all treatment is to enable children with asthma to lead absolutely normal lives and all but a small minority are able to do so. Your first source of help should be your GP. Because asthma in children is so common many GP surgeries run special 'asthma clinics' with specially trained asthma nurses. If yours doesn't it might be worth finding a local practice which does. Childhood asthma should be regularly monitored to make sure prescribed treatments continue to work effectively. Your GP or the asthma nurse will let you know how often to take your child for a check-up.

Asthma treatments usually come in the form of **inhalers**. There are two basic kinds, **relievers** and **preventers**. Your GP will usually prescribe reliever medication first, to see if that is enough to control the symptoms. If it isn't, then preventer medication will also be prescribed.

The drugs used to relieve asthma symptoms are called **bronchodilators**. As the name suggests, they work by relaxing the muscles surrounding the air passages in the lungs and are usually effective within minutes. Two of the most common bronchodilators are salbutamol (Ventolin) and terbutaline (Bricanyl). Your GP or practice nurse will show you and your child how to use the inhaler. With very young children a **spacer** – a clear plastic device looking rather like a water-bottle – and/or **mask** might be needed, too, to ensure that enough of the medication is inhaled at one puff.

Most children learn to use their inhaler very quickly and without any difficulty, and of course it's important that your child gets used to this form of treatment and is happy using it. Other reliever medications are available, so if you are not happy with the treatment your child gets, or it doesn't seem to be effective at controlling her symptoms, your doctor will be able to offer a more suitable alternative.

Quite often, reliever medication on its own is not enough to control asthma symptoms. In this case, **preventer** medication will also be prescribed. This usually comes in the form of corticosteroid drugs with names like beclomethazone (Becotide and Becloforte), budesonide (Pulmicort) and fluticazone (Flixotide). Preventer medication is also inhaled, though the inhalers are usually brown, white, orange or red, unlike the blue reliever inhalers. Preventer drugs are designed to be taken twice a day, whether or not asthma symptoms are present. Corticosteroids reduce inflammation, so that the airways are less likely to flare up when they come across an asthma trigger. The effect builds up over a few days, so it's important to keep taking them.

Parents are naturally concerned about treating children with drugs, particularly steroids. Corticosteroids, however, have an excellent safety record and are not to be confused with the anabolic steroids taken by body-builders.

Most childhood asthma can be controlled by a combination of preventer and reliever medication, plus avoidance, as far as possible, of the **triggers** which bring on asthma attacks. These are different for every child and it's only by experience that you learn which

13

triggers affect your child most. Common asthma triggers include:

- colds and other respiratory infections – most children's asthma is worse when they get a cold, and the symptoms can linger for weeks;
- animal dander – the mixture of pet hair and saliva shed around the home by furry or feathery creatures;
- house-dust mites – tiny creatures which live and breed in our warm, modern homes, especially in bedding, carpets and soft furnishings;
- passive smoking – children whose parents smoke inhale the equivalent of 60–150 cigarettes' worth of chemicals a year;
- exercise – exercise can bring on asthma attacks, though it is obviously important that children with asthma are able to run around and play like other children. Breathlessness after exercise in young children should always be investigated. Usually, once your child has been prescribed an inhaler, a puff or two of reliever medication should enable him to take part in school sports, etc. If it doesn't, perhaps the medication needs adjusting;
- stress, excitement or worry can sometimes bring on an attack;
- cold air – a puff of an inhaler plus a scarf round the face can help;
- other, less common triggers include food allergies (see Chapter 4) or a reaction to another kind of medication. Always tell your doctor or pharmacist that your child is asthmatic.

Some teenage girls find that their asthma is affected by their menstrual cycle and are advised to adjust their 'preventer' medication at those times of the month.

The message from health professionals is that the vast majority of cases of childhood asthma can be controlled with a combination of inhalers. In rare or more severe cases, steroid tablets may be prescribed for a short time.

Lifestyle adjustments, such as replacing carpets with wooden floors, fabric seats with leather and curtains with blinds, avoiding pets and smoking in the home, using hypo-allergenic bedding and vacuum cleaners with special air filters, can sometimes be helpful. Contact Asthma UK (address on p. 87) for advice on these issues as they have access to the most up-to-date research. However, you can't keep your child in a sterile bubble and you always need to strike a balance between avoiding the worst asthma triggers and allowing your child to take part in the normal activities of everyday life.

What to do in case of an asthma attack

Everyone with whom your child comes into contact should know what to do in case of an asthma attack – friends, family, babysitters, teachers, playgroup leaders, Guide or Scout captains. Advice from Asthma UK is:

• stay calm and reassuring;
• don't put your arm round the child as this is constricting;
• give him his reliever (blue) inhaler, using a spacer if he has one;
• encourage him to breathe slowly and evenly, sitting in an upright position.

The reliever should start to work in five to ten minutes. If it does not, or the child seems exhausted or so upset he is unable to speak, call the doctor or an ambulance. If a child has an attack while out and about and doesn't seem to be responding to his normal medication, don't hesitate to take him to the nearest A&E department.

Asthma in schools

Great progress has been made in the last ten years towards including children with asthma in all normal childhood experiences, including pre-school and school. Asthma UK has booklets about asthma management in school which parents and teachers will find helpful. Both the National Childminding Association (contact details on p. 88) and the Pre-School Learning Alliance (contact details on p. 88) can offer advice on looking after small children with asthma, including:

• agreements between parents and carers on administering medication;
• where and how inhalers are looked after;
• avoiding asthma triggers in the environment – for instance, pet-free homes and nurseries, no-smoking policies;
• what to do in an emergency.

In 1996, the Department for Education and Skills and the Department of Health issued a set of guidelines called *Supporting Children with Medical Needs*, designed to help schools formulate a policy for including children with asthma – and other chronic medical conditions like diabetes – in all normal school activities. Asthma UK

15

can also supply a Schools Pack, which has details of the condition, information about what to do when a student with asthma joins the class, emergency instructions and possible discussion topics for classroom work on asthma.

Whether your child is in primary or secondary school, it's vital that all her teachers know that she has asthma and carries an inhaler. It's recommended that all but the very smallest children should be allowed to have their inhaler with them at all times, and that it should be clearly labelled with their name. The child's class teacher, the head, year tutor or another appropriate member of staff should also have a labelled, spare inhaler in case of emergencies. Parents are normally expected to give the school written permission to administer medication where necessary.

Again, it's wise to have a chat to your child's class teacher and explain which factors could trigger an asthma attack. If your child is likely to be sensitive to certain cookery ingredients or fumes from the science lab, this is the time to raise your concerns. Having asthma, though, should not be an excuse for your child to be excused PE or games lessons (unless, of course, he or she is really ill). Manchester United star Paul Scholes and international long-distance runner Paula Radcliffe are both asthma sufferers, and all children, including asthmatic children, need to keep fit!

Forms are available from the Department of Education and Skills for you and the school to fill in so that a Healthcare Plan can be formulated for your child. Once this is done, everyone knows exactly what their responsibilities are.

Specialist asthma nurses advise parents

- to make sure their child's asthma is regularly monitored so that he is always receiving the right medication;
- to make sure he understands what his preventer and reliever inhalers are for and how to use them;
- that he keeps them with him at all times;
- that his school has a properly formulated asthma policy and that all his teachers know that he has asthma.

What about the future?

Parents frequently ask whether their asthmatic child is likely to grow out of the condition. Some children undoubtedly do; asthma is said to affect between 10 and 20 per cent of British children and only about 5 to 10 per cent of adults, according to British Lung Foundation figures. Long-term medical studies indicate that just under half of all Britons have experienced at least one wheezy episode before they reach middle age.

However, it's not possible to predict with certainty whether a particular child will outgrow his or her asthma. There seems to be a tendency for those whose asthma is mild to grow out of it, whereas those more seriously affected seem more likely to continue having respiratory problems in later life. More young boys have asthma than young girls, but in adolescence girls tend to catch up. By the age of 18 slightly more young women than young men are affected by the condition.

Teenagers should be encouraged to take responsibility for their own health, including asthma management. Teens with asthma have an excellent excuse to resist peer pressure to smoke! Asthma UK's literature is clearly written and easy to follow and might be more acceptable to teens than advice from Mum and Dad. They also have a website, <**www.kickasthma.org.uk**>, aimed specifically at teen-agers. Once they are old enough to go away to university it can be hard for parents to hand over complete responsibility. The Anaphylaxis Campaign (contact details on p. 87) has an excellent booklet, *Letting Go – Teaching an Allergic Child Responsibility*, which is appropriate for youngsters with asthma as well as other allergic conditions.

Could complementary therapies help?

Asthma UK is open-minded about the use of complementary therapies to treat asthma, and can send out factsheets on the subject. They do, however, make the point that no reputable complementary therapist will recommend throwing away your child's inhalers. As is so often the case, there are few double-blind, placebo-controlled clinical trials of complementary therapies and their effectiveness in treating the condition. However, there is anecdotal evidence that some children find herbal medicine, acupuncture, and 'breathing' therapies like yoga and Buteyko – a regime of breathing exercises devised by a Russian professor more than fifty years ago – helpful.

'If I'm doing my job properly, a child's need for inhalers should lessen,' said one qualified medical herbalist, who has treated her own daughter's asthma with some success.

If approaching any complementary practitioner you should make sure they are properly trained, qualified and registered with a reputable professional body such as the National Institute of Medical Herbalists or the Acupuncture Council (contact details on pp. 95 and 94). It is also worth remembering that some complementary medicines are definitely *unsuitable* for anyone with asthma or a related allergic condition. Royal Jelly and Propolis, products produced by bees and marketed as health supplements, have sometimes produced severe allergic reactions and, in Australia at least, now carry a health warning that they are not suitable for people with asthma.

A cure for asthma?

At the moment it doesn't seem likely that a cure for asthma will be found in the next few years, although research is ongoing. The rise in obesity among children is worrying asthma specialists, since asthma is known to be commoner among heavier children and those with the condition are often advised to try to lose weight. Work is being done on prevention, even looking at the effect of maternal diet, so that in future doctors may be able to advise mums-to-be which foods might have a protective effect. There are studies taking place on the relationships between the Pill and asthma and paracetamol and asthma, since the rise in childhood asthma cases has coincided with an increase in the use of paracetamol-based medicines for children, though no causal link has been found so far.

A research team at the National Heart and Lung Institute in London is working on possible vaccines against cat allergy, house-dust mite allergy and pollen allergy which might benefit many asthmatics for whom these are triggers. Researchers are also hoping to refine and improve treatments, especially the treatment of very young children who wheeze, as they don't respond very well to currently available medication.

3

Eczema

What is eczema?

The word 'eczema' is used to describe a number of conditions affecting the skin. Some children have a very mild form of eczema which just means their skin tends to be dry and flaky and needs special care. In more serious cases, eczema leads to soreness, unbearable itching, inflammation, and the formation of dry, crusty patches and blisters which may 'weep' or bleed when scratched.

Other terms that may be used in describing eczema are:

- **dermatitis** – which is another word for eczema;
- **atopic eczema** – the most common form of childhood eczema; it's linked with other allergic conditions like asthma and hay fever and often runs in families;
- **allergic contact dermatitis**, which occurs when the skin comes into contact with a substance which causes an allergic reaction; rubber, glues and some chemicals can all cause allergic reactions in sensitive children;
- **irritant contact dermatitis/eczema**, caused by contact with substances which irritate the skin, such as harsh detergents;
- **seborrhoeic eczema**, which starts with an itchy, scaly scalp and dandruff and can spread to other parts of the body. Babies often get a version of this known as cradle cap. It looks unpleasant but is not especially troublesome and most babies grow out of it without special treatment.

Other forms of eczema may involve itchy blisters which appear on the fingers and soles of the feet, or coin-shaped patches on the arms and legs. Another, rare form of eczema seems to be caused by exposure to the sun's ultra-violet rays.

According to the National Eczema Society, eczema now affects as many as one fifth of British schoolchildren. Like other allergic conditions, it seems to be becoming more common, although exactly why this should be is not completely understood. The words 'eczema' and 'dermatitis' mean the same thing. Many children with eczema suffer from dry, itchy and inflamed skin which weeps and bleeds, particularly if they are tempted to scratch it. Some babies are actually born with dry skin, but most commonly eczema begins to develop in babies from about six weeks old and can continue to affect them throughout their childhood. The good news is that many children – perhaps three-quarters of all those affected – grow out of the condition around the time of puberty. Again, the reasons for this are not known.

Eczema affects different children differently. It often appears first of all on the baby's face, scalp or nappy area and can then spread to the rest of the body.

Eczema is not contagious – in other words, it isn't something that children can 'catch' or spread to other children. It often runs in families, usually families where other allergic conditions like asthma and hay fever also exist. Many children suffer from eczema in addition to other allergic-type reactions.

How the skin works

The skin is the largest organ in the body and receives about a third of the blood pumped from the heart. It's there to regulate body heat and water loss, to protect us from the sun and to help us get rid of waste products. An adult's skin covers an area of 1.75 square metres and makes up about 7 per cent of total body weight. Human skin is constantly renewing itself and it's estimated that the whole skin is replaced every three weeks.

The skin has three layers:

The **epidermis**, or outer layer, is the body's first line of defence against injury. As skin cells grow older they work their way up to the surface of the skin, where they gradually die off and are shed, a process we don't normally notice.

The **dermis**, the next layer, produces lubrication and is also elastic, allowing the skin to stretch as we grow. Sweat glands are found in this layer.

Beneath these two layers is a layer of **subcutaneous fat** which acts as insulation, keeping us warm when it's cold and allowing heat loss when it's hot.

A healthy skin needs to be moist to remain supple and elastic. Many factors dry out the skin – from the normal process of ageing to not drinking enough water. In childhood eczema the skin is particularly dry, flaky and sore. Scratching makes the itching worse, and cracked, split or bleeding skin is also extremely vulnerable to bacterial infections.

What causes eczema?

We don't know why some allergy-prone children develop eczema. However, when a child has a tendency to the condition, a flare-up can be caused by all kinds of things, from stress to environmental factors like house-dust mites, pet dander, wool and other fabrics, household chemicals which may irritate the skin, food allergy, or even sudden changes in temperature or humidity.

The problems living with eczema can cause

Eczema is not life-threatening, but it can have a huge effect on the quality of life of not only the child but his or her whole family.

'My son had his first bath at two days old and came out looking like a beetroot,' says Sandie, whose 5-year-old has very severe eczema.

'It started on his scalp but soon spread to his whole body. He spent a year being treated with strong steroids, which worked well but made him put on weight. He was also a very poor sleeper.'

Sandie's doctors showed her how to 'wet-wrap' her small son, a technique often used to control the constant itching. The child's body is covered with greasy emollients, plus steroid cream if necessary, and then wrapped in warm-water bandages topped with dry ones so that he looks like a mummy.

'If his skin was allowed to dry out, the eczema became a lot worse,' says Sandie.

The bandages help his skin to absorb all the cream and mean that he can't scratch. I would have to wake him at 11.30 and then again at 4.30 in the morning to spray him with warm water. Although it did help his skin, it meant that we were both constantly exhausted. Before I began wet-wrapping I would have to change his sheets three times a night anyway because he would scratch his skin until it bled.

Just about everything we do is ruled by Alex's eczema and other allergies. He has a little pot of emollient cream that he carries to school so that he can use it when he needs to, and dispensers around the house so that he can help himself. Hospital tests have shown that Alex is allergic to cats and dogs, which we already knew because his face swells up and his eyes close if he goes into a home where there's a pet in the house. He doesn't have to touch them for this to happen to him. Grass pollen, house-dust mites and some household chemicals have the same effect and he uses an inhaler for his asthma. I have to carry a large handbag everywhere we go, with his inhalers and spacer and emollient and anti-histamines.

The itch–scratch cycle

People who are unaffected by eczema can only begin to imagine how irritating and distressing having constantly itchy skin can be. It's the hardest part of living with eczema. Constantly telling children not to scratch because they will only make their skin feel worse doesn't really help, so what can be done to control that maddening itch?

The National Eczema Society (contact details on p. 87) has lots of helpful tips. They point out, first of all, that scratching is a natural response to itching, but that it makes skin which is already sore and sensitive even more sore. Often it's the scratching, rather than the condition itself, which breaks the skin and makes it bleed. Once the skin is broken, the skin is at greater risk of infection and also of reacting to allergens like pollen, soaps and any household chemicals.

Itching can be made worse by

- changes in temperature – for instance, in bed at night;
- sweating after sport or exercise;
- fabrics like wool, rough seams and loose threads on clothing;
- irritant substances like pollen and pet dander;
- stress and tiredness. As children with eczema are often poor sleepers this can be a vicious circle.

Itching can be helped by

- using plenty of emollients on the child's skin, smoothed in gently;
- patting the skin dry after a bath;
- wearing cotton gloves or mittens in bed;

- distracting the child with toys and games;
- placing a well-wrapped bag of frozen peas on the itchy area;
- keeping cool and dressing the child in layers which can be adjusted as the temperature changes;
- making sure the child's condition is regularly monitored in case his treatments need changing.

Can eczema be cured?

At present there is no cure for eczema. However, like other allergic conditions, it can be managed so that most affected children are able to enjoy a near-normal life, certainly in between flare-ups. Most cases of childhood eczema seem to respond quite well to the range of treatments now available. There are also lifestyle adjustments you can make which may help – for example, always dressing your child in cotton clothing, buying anti-allergy bedding to protect against contact with house-dust mites, and keeping your home cool.

Most cases of childhood eczema are treated with a combination of **emollients** and **topical steroids**. Emollients are basically moisturizers which, when applied several times a day, will form a protective layer over the skin and reduce the dryness. They are available as creams, ointments, lotions, 'soaps' and medicinal bath oils. Some are obtainable directly from your pharmacist, others on prescription only. E45 and Oilatum are among the best known. E45 has a special children's range called E45 Junior, and Oilatum also do a Junior Bath Formula and cream emollient.

Corticosteroids, as steroids are sometimes known, are derived from, or are synthetic variants of, the natural hormones which are produced in the upper part, or cortex, of the adrenal glands. Corticosteroid drugs are normally used to control inflammation, especially the inflammation caused by inappropriate reactions of the immune system. Topical steroids are specially designed to be used on the skin. They come as creams, ointments or lotions, in a variety of strengths or 'potencies'. Your child's doctor will prescribe whichever strength seems most appropriate. Topical steroids can usually bring skin conditions like eczema under control quite quickly. If your child's skin improves after a short course of steroids, you may then be able to control the symptoms with emollients alone, or with a less potent steroid.

Parents are often, understandably, concerned about treating children with potent steroids. Sometimes this is because of concern about possible side-effects, and sometimes because they are confused with the anabolic steroids – related to male sex hormones – used illegally by body-builders and other athletes to increase muscle bulk and body growth.

All drugs, including topical steroids, carry the risk of side-effects. Over-use of steroids can sometimes lead to thinning of the skin. However, they have been in use for treating childhood eczema for thirty years and have a good general safety record. Like all medicines they should be used carefully and according to the doctor's instructions about how much and how often to use them. Without steroids, a child with severe eczema may end up with long-term skin damage. There is, of course, always the possibility that your child will react badly to a particular medication. If this happens, your doctor will be able to prescribe an alternative.

Dr Frances Lawlor, a dermatologist working in East London, says that she is able to reassure worried parents that steroids are safe to use.

'Some parents have not been shown or told how to use them properly,' she comments. 'These days, with different preparations available for use on different parts of the body and treatment being prescribed for an appropriate length of time, we rarely see any problems.'

Frequent **bathing** is also recommended for children with eczema, although, to avoid any drying effects, special bath oils should be added to the bath water which should be warm, neither too hot nor too cold.

A special light treatment, called **PUVA** (which stands for Psoralen and Ultra-Violet Light) can be used to treat those with severe eczema if emollients and steroids don't seem to be effective. Dr Lawlor says that this may be useful for older children only, as it involves standing still in front of a light box for longer than most small children would be able to tolerate.

Another possibility in cases of severe eczema which haven't responded to standard treatments is the use of the immunosuppressant drug **cyclosporin**.

'It's easy to take and effective in some cases,' comments Dr Lawlor, 'but not very popular with children because they have to have regular blood tests, which most children don't like.'

Other treatments offered may include **anti-histamines** to relieve the itching and help children sleep, or **antibiotics** to clear up any infection.

Diet and eczema

According to Allergy UK, about 15 per cent of childhood eczema is food-related. If you suspect that your child's skin problems are triggered by certain foods, the best thing to do is to ask to be referred to an allergist so that proper skin and blood tests can be carried out. (See Chapter 4 for more information on food allergy and intolerance.) The National Eczema Society points out that diet is unlikely to be the only factor involved if your child has eczema. Only a small number of children with eczema are likely to be helped by a change of diet.

In some children, the effect of eating a particular food is very obvious. The child's itching becomes worse and there is redness, swelling and irritation around the mouth. Skin symptoms like urticaria (nettle rash) and swelling can appear from five minutes to two hours after eating the food.

The usual tests for food allergy – so-called 'skin prick tests' or 'RAST (blood) tests' – can be given to children whose eczema seems to be brought on by foods. However, they are not 100 per cent reliable, especially in very young children. The only way to find out if a food is a trigger is to exclude it from the child's diet for two to six weeks, then slowly re-introduce it to see if the symptoms recur. Exclusion diets like this should only be undertaken under the supervision of a dietician.

Lifestyle changes

The sort of lifestyle changes recommended for all allergic children and their families may benefit those with eczema too. Allergen avoidance can help, but in order to identify the allergens which affect your child it is best to take advice from an allergy expert. Replacing your carpets with wooden floors, your upholstered furniture with leather or wicker seating, and buying anti-allergy products can be an expensive business. You need to be sure you are helping your child before embarking on a lot of changes.

Tony and Andrea's 6-year-old daughter Amber has had severe eczema since she was four months old. It is now well controlled with emollients and potent steroids. Tony and Andrea have also done everything they can to ensure that their home is as allergen-free as possible. They are non-smokers and have no pets. Tony says,

We don't have any carpets or curtains, and we have bought special anti-dust-mite bedding for Amber. The household products we use are all perfume-free. The Eczema Society magazine carries adverts for lots of products and they are not too hard to find as so many families need them these days.

Amber's clothes need to be 100 per cent cotton or silk. She has special sleep-suits with mittens called 'Cotton Comfort' so that we can cover her in emollient at night and put her straight into her sleep-suit. They even have seams and labels on the outside so they don't cause any irritation. They're quite expensive, but worth it. Amber also has a portable air-conditioner in her room and we have pollen filters in our car.

Eczema in schools

As soon as children are old enough to go to playgroup, nursery or school, parents can find themselves explaining to teachers, pupils and other parents what eczema is and how it can affect their child. The Eczema Society has a Schools Pack that can be helpful as it emphasizes that eczema

- is not catching;
- is nothing to do with poor personal hygiene.

It's important for parents and teacher to get together so that the teacher – who may have worked with children with eczema before, but needs to know how it affects *your* child – has a clear idea of how the condition is managed. For instance, it helps if the teacher knows

- how much time your child is likely to need for hospital appointments, etc.;
- what sort of treatment the child has and how long it takes;
- what triggers a flare-up and which school activities may cause

problems – for instance, painting, playing with sand and water, hand-washing, getting too hot or cold;
• if your child sleeps badly and is likely to be very tired/irritable in school.

Parents report variable degrees of co-operation from their children's schools. Some are clearly more sympathetic than others. Sandie's son Alex has asthma as well as eczema and she says that his school considers her a 'neurotic mum'.

He wasn't included when his class went on a trip to a local farm, and when I offered to go and help they just said brusquely that they didn't need my help. The other children play about with his creams and emollients and he keeps picking up tummy bugs because it's hard for him to wash and dry his hands after using the toilet. His hands are quite badly affected and the other children don't want to hold hands with him. He did once say he wished he had normal skin but he has never known anything different.

By contrast, 6-year-old Amber has had plenty of support from her nursery and primary school.
'The head said they have another child with peanut allergy and one who can't eat eggs, and they were happy to work out an action plan for Amber,' says her mum Andrea.

It's obvious Amber has eczema as it's all over her hands and face, but she is friendly and bubbly and mixes well with other children. She does gym and swimming and isn't self-conscious about people seeing her. If I hear any whispers I will explain or Amber will tell them, 'It's just my tickly skin!'

There are ways round most of the difficulties that can arise. For example, your child may be able to sit in a shady seat away from the window, wear a cotton vest under his nylon football shirt, wear cotton gloves for art work, and keep a towel and soap substitutes in the cloakroom so that she doesn't have to use school soap and paper towels which may irritate sore, sensitive skin.

Like any children who are seen as 'different', children with eczema can sometimes be bullied or made to feel that they are the odd ones out. This is something that both teachers and parents

27

should be aware of. All schools are supposed to have anti-bullying strategies in place and physical and mental cruelty should not be tolerated. Children should know that their concerns are taken seriously by both parents and teachers.

Teenagers and eczema

Many children grow out of childhood eczema at puberty. For those who don't, the teenage years can be difficult. Changing schools, from primary school where a child is taught by one teacher who is familiar with her condition, to secondary school where she is taught by several different teachers and has to meet dozens of new schoolmates, can be traumatic. It's a good idea for parents to meet school staff so that arrangements can be made to deal with any problems that may arise. Flexibility on the part of the school makes life easier for all concerned. Stress can make eczema worse so exam times are especially difficult for affected youngsters.

According to the National Eczema Society (NES), 86 per cent of teenagers polled said they felt self-conscious about their condition. At an age when appearance really matters and young people are beginning to take an interest in the opposite sex, having a severe skin problem can affect their self-esteem. The NES has a helpful leaflet, *Live your Life – Information for Teenagers with Eczema*, with down-to-earth advice aimed at helping teenagers to take control of their lives, rather than letting their condition 'take over'. The leaflet points out that nobody is perfect – even the stunning models and pop stars in magazines and on TV have had their blemishes airbrushed out – and that friends worth having are those who respond to you as a whole person and love you for who you are.

They recommend that young people with eczema:

- take up new challenges and interests and find things they're good at;
- exercise regularly so that they are in good health;
- hang round with people who make them feel good about themselves;
- take control of their own skincare regime, avoiding irritants and keeping the skin well moisturized;
- learn a relaxation technique such as meditation, yoga or t'ai chi;

- recognize when they need practical or emotional support. As well as confiding in family and friends, they can talk to a youth counsellor or contact Changing Faces (contact details on p. 95).

Complementary therapies

As with most conditions for which modern science has not yet found a cure, it is sometimes tempting to look outside conventional medicine for help. The National Eczema Society stresses that anyone contemplating using any 'alternative' therapy should check with their GP and also make sure that the therapist they consult is qualified, experienced and a member of a recognized professional organization. Some complementary therapists recommend that patients stop using their prescribed medication, which can have distressing results. It is also worth remembering that few complementary therapies have undergone the range of double-blind, placebo-controlled clinical trials necessary before conventional drug treatments come on to the market. You can't assume that because something is 'natural', plant- or herb-based, that it is harmless. There are plenty of natural poisons, as well as herbal preparations which react badly with other medications, both conventional and complementary.

Having said all that, there have been some trials in recent years of Chinese herbal medicines as a treatment for eczema. The NES says that results were encouraging but that anyone contemplating using Chinese herbs should be carefully monitored by their GP. Not all Chinese herbal preparations are made from standardized ingredients, and some creams prescribed by Chinese practitioners have been found to contain steroids.

Therapies which promote relaxation, such as hypnotherapy, which has been used on young eczema patients at Great Ormond Street Hospital, can help children feel more comfortable and in control, even though it won't cure their eczema.

4

Food allergy

'The diagnosis of food allergy is one of the most difficult areas in medicine.' That's a direct quote from an Allergy UK leaflet and illustrates how hard it can be to work out whether your child's problem is caused by a food allergy, and if it is, which food is causing the problem.

In 2001 the British Nutrition Foundation (BNF) was so concerned about the number of people – about a fifth of the entire population – claiming to have food allergies that it commissioned a report, *Adverse Reactions to Food*. The Foundation said that with a variety of health problems from upset stomachs to spots to migraine being blamed on 'food allergy' the public was sometimes being given 'inappropriate and sometimes dangerous' dietary advice.

The BNF claims that food **intolerance** – an adverse reaction to a food or ingredient – affects about 5–8 per cent of children, and food **allergy** – an adverse reaction to food involving the immune system – affects no more than 1–2 per cent of children. Like other allergic conditions, food allergies tend to run in families, which is why pregnant women who are aware of allergic conditions like asthma and hay fever in their own and their partners' families are advised to watch their diet during pregnancy and avoid common allergens like peanuts and peanut products. Guidelines from the Department of Health recommend that babies should be breast- or bottle-fed until they are four months old, and that solid foods should be introduced as follows:

- at 4–6 months – rice, meat, chicken, pulses, vegetables, fruit (but not citrus fruit);
- at 6–12 months – wheat-based foods like bread and biscuits, fish, eggs, yogurt, cheese, citrus fruit;
- at 12 months plus – ordinary cow's milk.

It's also suggested that children should not be given peanuts or peanut products like peanut butter until they are at least a year old, and over 5 in families where there are peanut or other allergies.

Carina Venter, Allergy Research Dietician at the David Hide Asthma and Allergy Research Centre on the Isle of Wight, makes similar recommendations to the parents of children referred to her.

'If possible, babies should be breast-fed exclusively for at least four months and preferably six months,' she says.

Mothers of high-risk infants (from atopic families) may wish to avoid eating peanuts while they are breast-feeding. If an alternative to breast milk is needed, choose a low-allergy formula. Soy, goat or cow's milk formula or off-the-shelf cow's, goat's, sheep's, soy or rice milks should not be given.

Solids should not be given before four months, ideally not before six months. I recommend starting with low-allergenic foods like rice, potatoes, root and green vegetables, apple, pear, banana and stone fruit.

From six months, all foods can be introduced. Wheat, egg, chicken, cow's milk, fish, oranges, peas and tomatoes should be introduced singly and with caution, no more than one new allergenic food per week. It may be wise to introduce well-cooked egg before giving your baby runny egg, for example egg 'soldiers'.

The small quantity of soy present in foods like bread and commercial baby-food is acceptable from six months, and by the time your baby is a year old all the major high-risk foods should have been introduced apart from peanuts.

New mothers having problems with breast-feeding should contact their midwife or health visitor for advice, or alternatively get in touch with the National Childbirth Trust (contact details on p. 87).

Living with food allergy is difficult because, unlike other allergens, you can't avoid food! It's especially important that growing children are able to eat a healthy, balanced diet containing foods from all the major food groups – carbohydrates, protein, some fats, fruit and vegetables and fibre. Any food which has to be excluded from the diet because of an allergy needs to be replaced by something that can give the child the same amount of nourishment. This is why the parents of children with food allergies are advised to consult a paediatric dietician before making the decision to put their child on an 'exclusion' diet.

Common food allergies in children

The commonest food allergies in children are to cow's milk, eggs, wheat, soya, peanuts, tree nuts, fish and shellfish, and some fruits. Symptoms of food allergy vary from child to child and can also vary in the degree of severity. They can include facial swelling and flushing, a blotchy, itchy rash, a feeling that the throat is swelling up, breathing difficulties, wheezing, nausea and vomiting, colic or diarrhoea. The most serious form of food allergy causes anaphylaxis (see Chapter 5) which affects the whole body and can, if untreated, prove fatal. These reactions normally occur very soon after eating the offending food, as the child's immune system recognizes the substance and releases histamines into the body.

Some childhood food allergies disappear after a year or two. For example, the majority of children allergic to cow's milk have grown out of it by the age of about 3, and most by the time they are old enough for school. Egg intolerance is also associated with early childhood. Peanut allergy, by contrast, tends to be a life-long problem. The reasons for this are not yet known.

There is also what is known as 'oral allergy syndrome' where certain fruits and vegetables can cause itching and/or rashes around the mouth and lips. These sometimes occur in pollen-sensitive children (see Chapter 6) because the same proteins are found in some pollens. Children who react to ragweed pollen may also react to melon, and children who are sensitive to birch pollen may have the same reaction to apples. Cooked fruit may not cause the same reaction.

Lactose intolerance

Lactose intolerance, which occurs in older children and adults, is not, strictly speaking, an allergy, since the immune system is not involved. Children with the condition suffer from stomach pain and diarrhoea if they drink a lot of milk, though small amounts may be tolerated without problems. This is because their bodies do not produce enough of the enzyme lactase, which digests lactose, the natural sugar found in milk. Other dairy products like cheese and yogurt may cause fewer problems, and lactose-reduced milks can be found in health-food stores.

There have been suggestions that some of the 'colicky' babies who cry a lot in their first three months of life may actually be suffering from something called 'transient lactose intolerance'. A double-blind, placebo-controlled study carried out at Guy's Hospital in London in 2001 looked at 53 babies with colic. It found that although there does not seem to be one single cause of colic in all babies, adding a lactase enzyme to babies' feed reduced crying time and distress by 45 per cent.

Coeliac disease

Coeliac disease is caused by sensitivity to gluten and is estimated to affect one person in 200 in Britain. The true incidence is still not known, according to support group Coeliac UK, and there are probably thousands of people who are still undiagnosed. It isn't, strictly speaking, an allergy, but a bowel disease caused by damage to the **villi**, finger-like projections in the lining of the small intestine. (The word 'coeliac' comes from the Greek word *koiliakos* which means suffering of the bowels.)

Gluten is the protein found in wheat, rye and barley. The exact mechanism by which gluten damages the small intestine is not yet known. Children with coeliac disease can't tolerate gluten in any form. Symptoms are usually first noticed at the time of weaning, when wheat is first introduced into the baby's diet. The baby may suffer from diarrhoea, irritability and 'failure to thrive'. Undiagnosed coeliac disease in children can stunt their growth and have an impact on their development. However, once coeliac disease is diagnosed and gluten removed from the diet, the symptoms disappear.

In most cases, it's a lifelong condition and it's necessary for the child to continue to follow a gluten-free diet. As wheat is such a staple food in Britain, following a wheat-free diet might seem a bit daunting at first. It's not only present in basics like bread and pasta, but also as a filler in everything from soup and sauces to sausages. Studying food labels is not always helpful because terms like 'modified starch' or 'vegetable protein' may be used. A strict gluten-free diet will also involve using separate toasters and breadboards and avoiding bakery products which may be contaminated with gluten-containing items. Even chip-shop chips may have been fried in the same fat used for gluten-containing batter!

However, shopping for a gluten-free diet is easier than it used to be. Many supermarkets and health-food stores now stock a range of gluten-free products, and specialist manufacturers produce whole ranges of gluten-free foods. Many common foods like fruit, rice, potatoes, vegetables, meat and milk are naturally gluten-free, and most coeliacs can tolerate oat products without harm. Gluten-free cookery books are also available. For more information, contact Coeliac UK (contact details on p. 89).

Some children and teenagers with coeliac disease also develop a skin inflammation called dermatitis herpetiformis or DH, which causes small, itchy blisters to form on their elbows, forearms, buttocks and knees, or indeed anywhere on the body. Children with DH test positive for coeliac disease though they may have none of the characteristic symptoms of 'failure to thrive' and diarrhoea. DH can be treated with drugs and a gluten-free diet is also recommended.

Obtaining a diagnosis

Your GP will, of course, be your first port of call if you want to find out whether your child has a food allergy and which food might be causing it. Obtaining a diagnosis is not always easy. You can help your doctor by letting her know

- whether there are allergic disorders like asthma or eczema in the family;
- whether the same symptoms occur each time your child eats a particular food;
- exactly what the symptoms are – whether your child has breathing problems, develops a rash, or suffers from an upset stomach;
- whether you have tried cutting the food out of your child's diet and whether this helped.

If it looks as though your child has an allergy your GP should be able to refer you to a specialist. However, the Royal College of Physicians' report in June 2003, *Allergy – the Unmet Need*, found that NHS provision for allergy testing was patchy at best. Most allergy specialists are based in London and the South East, and there is only one consultant allergist for every 2 million of the UK

it with potato, corn or rice. As a dietician, I will ensure the child's diet has plenty of different tastes and textures. If I'm concerned about a specific nutrient like calcium or iron, I will provide parents with a list of foods with a high iron or calcium content.

Help outside the home

It can also be difficult to convince everyone else that the child is not just being faddy – it *matters* that she is not given foods she can't tolerate. You can watch her diet at home, but what happens when she goes to playgroup, nursery or school, or when she is invited to children's parties?

The increased incidence of childhood allergies means that most childminders, playgroup leaders, nursery nurses and teachers are used to making arrangements for children on special diets. It's important that everyone who cares for your child, including dinner ladies and babysitters, knows what she can and can't eat. It's often easiest to provide your child with a suitable packed lunch. Quite small children are often co-operative when they know they must not eat certain foods 'because it makes me poorly'.

Shopping with a food allergy

As in the case of coeliac disease, mainstream manufacturers, supermarkets and specialist food producers have made food-buying for the allergic child much easier than it used to be. Most supermarkets have their special 'Free From' ranges, and food labels often tell you whether a product is, or is not, suitable for those with the most common allergies. You'll need to familiarize yourself with the terms used in food labelling such as 'starch' or 'hydrolysed vegetable protein'.

For example, if your child is on a dairy-free diet, that means cutting out obvious dairy products like butter, cheese and yogurt. Alternatives are often available in supermarkets as well as specialist shops, in the form of soya milks and desserts. When reading food labels, you will also have to avoid items containing casein, caseinates, hydrolysed casein, sodium caseinate, lactose and whey, which are all derived from milk.

If the label doesn't make it clear, you can usually obtain help from

Customer Services in the form of leaflets (for contact details see p. 90). Major supermarkets and food manufacturers should be able to tell you which of their products are suitable for children on exclusion or restricted diets.

There are also specialist manufacturers, whose products are available either in supermarkets or health-food stores. Hull-based company Baker's Delight (contact details on p. 90) is one of several producers of a range of wheat- and gluten-free bread and cakes. *Allergy* magazine, the glossy sent out to supporters of Allergy UK and now also available from newsagents and supermarkets, has pages of advertisements for companies producing gluten-free, egg-free, dairy-free and other specialist products. Many of these companies offer free information and recipe booklets to customers and potential customers. (There is a list of companies producing allergy-friendly foods on p. 90.)

Keen cooks can often adapt favourite recipes using suitable alternative ingredients, and a browse around the cookery section of your local bookshop will yield entire cookery books catering for special diets, some particularly focused on children's meals. Support groups like Allergy UK and Coeliac UK can also offer suggestions. Vegetarian and vegan societies (contact details on p. 89) and cookery books are good sources of help, as is the Internet.

A London-based organization called Foods Matter (contact details on p. 91) produces a monthly magazine of the same name which carries articles on the latest research findings as well as 'personal experience' stories and tastings of new products. They also have an 'Allergy Agony Aunt' and a 'Find You a Doctor' service.

Food allergies and behavioural problems

For the past twenty or thirty years some experts have been suggesting that food allergy or intolerance may be a root cause of behavioural problems in children. Perhaps the best known of these is the late Dr Ben Feingold, formerly paediatrician and Chief Emeritus at the Kaiser Permanente Hospital in the USA. Dr Feingold's theory was that there was a link between food additives and conditions like hyperactivity or Attention Deficit Hyperactivity Disorder (ADHD), as it is now better known. Putting hyperactive children on a healthy diet, avoiding chemical additives and some natural foods containing salicylates (oranges, tomatoes, grapes and raisins, berry fruits) seemed to improve their behaviour problems in some cases.

In similar experiments in American young offenders' institutions, replacing the lads' diets of fast food and Coke with something healthier was said to improve anti-social behaviour and reduce re-offending. More recently, nutrition expert Patrick Holford in his book *Optimum Nutrition for the Mind* (Piatkus, 2003) quotes several studies of the effect of essential fatty acid supplements on children with ADHD and learning difficulties. One double-blind placebo-controlled trial of 41 8–12-year-olds, carried out at Oxford University, found that within 12 weeks the children taking the supplements did behave better.

In Britain, the Sussex-based Hyperactive Children's Support Group (HCSG) has been recommending dietary change as a way of managing ADHD since 1981. Mainstream medicine prefers to treat hyperactive children with stimulant medication like Ritalin and claims that there is little proof that a change in diet helps most children with ADHD.

Most recently a non-stimulant drug, Strattera (otherwise atomoxetine), has been licensed for the treatment of ADHD. Exactly how this works is not known, but six successful research studies have indicated that it is both safe and effective.

Some experts state bluntly that food intolerance does not cause ADHD (though it can make it worse) and that supplementing with vitamin B6 and zinc, as recommended by the HCSG, has not been proven to have any appreciable effect. Most recently, an American research study in 2003, reported in the *Alternative Medicine Review*, found that supplementing ADHD children's diet was just as effective as drugs as a way of improving their behaviour. A British study of 3-year-olds on the Isle of Wight, published in the journal *Archives of Disease in Childhood*, found that a high percentage of them were affected by food additives.

It does seem to be the case that a large proportion of hyperactive children come from atopic families, with a history of allergies like asthma and eczema, and also suffer from food intolerance. As well as food additives, many of the children in research studies reacted badly to cow's milk, eggs, wheat, chocolate, oranges and cheese. Parents do report fewer behavioural problems in children on the easy-to-follow diet recommended by the HCSG (contact details on p. 89).

Founder Sally Bunday, whose own son suffered from behaviour problems, poor sleep, asthma and continual catarrh until the family made dietary changes, says,

> Most parents find that artificial colourings cause most problems for their children, followed by certain preservatives, monosodium glutamate and aspartame. We have seen an Australian study which found that a mould retardant used in bread could also affect some children.
>
> Others react badly to salicylates, which are strong aspirin-like chemicals found in brightly coloured fruits like oranges.
>
> Food additives, cow's milk, chocolate, oranges and wheat are the most likely foods to cause difficulties. At the HCSG we feel that GPs should at least try to give dietary advice to the parents of children with behaviour problems and allergies.

At the very least, it can't do any harm to ensure your child eats the healthiest possible diet, free from artificial colourants and preservatives where possible.

5

Anaphylaxis

Most allergic conditions, while they can be uncomfortable and distressing, are not life-threatening. Anaphylaxis is at the extreme end of the allergy spectrum, a reaction which is so severe that, if untreated, it can kill. In cases of 'anaphylactic shock', after contact with even minute quantities of a particular allergen, the immune system reacts violently, producing large quantities of chemicals which can affect the whole body – including the skin, lungs and digestive organs. The blood pressure falls dramatically and the patient rapidly loses consciousness.

In 1993, 17-year-old Sarah Reading died after eating a slice of lemon meringue pie in a department store restaurant. The pie had contained traces of peanut, to which Sarah was fatally allergic. The following year the Anaphylaxis Campaign was set up by a group of parents including Sarah's father David, to provide help and advice to others whose children might be similarly affected, to press for better facilities for sufferers (including clearer food labelling) and to raise awareness of the condition among the medical community as well as the general public.

'Our aim now is to see that the Department of Health and Primary Care Trusts give anaphylaxis, and allergies generally, a much higher priority,' says David Reading.

Allergy is now a serious epidemic and, as the 2003 Royal College of Physicians' report showed, services for people with even life-threatening allergies are abysmal.

We are also working for much better awareness in the food industry and among restaurant staff. Currently, when severe reactions happen, it is often after the child has eaten in a restaurant or had a takeaway meal. Families have to rely on the assurances of the restaurant staff, and if they aren't sufficiently well informed, mistakes can be made.

Symptoms of anaphylaxis

These usually – but not always – come on very soon after exposure to the allergen and may include some of the following:

- itching or a strange metallic taste in the mouth;
- swelling of the throat and tongue;
- difficulty in breathing;
- difficulty in swallowing;
- skin rash (hives) anywhere on the body;
- flushed skin;
- stomach cramps, nausea and/or vomiting;
- increased heart rate;
- dizziness;
- feeling of sudden weakness;
- sense of doom;
- collapse and unconsciousness.

What are the causes?

Peanut allergy is perhaps the best known, and is becoming more common, in line with other allergic reactions. The reason for the increase is not yet known, though increased exposure to peanut products may help to explain it. Of the 8,000 members of the Anaphylaxis Campaign, 89 per cent have peanut allergy.

'Peanut allergy has tripled since the mid-1990s,' says David Reading. 'One in 200 young children used to be affected; now it is one in 70, so it is a very real increase.'

However, severely allergic children may react to almost any kind of food in this way. According to the Anaphylaxis Campaign, the most common triggers, in addition to peanuts, include other tree nuts like almonds, brazils, hazelnuts and walnuts, sesame seeds, shellfish, fish, eggs, dairy products, latex (natural rubber) and bee or wasp stings. Some drugs, like penicillin, can also cause anaphylactic reactions.

As anaphylaxis is part of the spectrum of allergic reactions, it is likely that many affected children will suffer from other allergic conditions too, for example asthma or eczema. The Anaphylaxis Campaign recommends that if your child has had a severe reaction to any food or substance, you should ask for him to be referred to an allergy specialist so that the allergy can be diagnosed and appropriate treatment prescribed. Small children with anaphylaxis can wear a badge saying so. Older children and teenagers can obtain a 'Medic-Alert' bracelet to wear, giving details of their condition and a 24-hour helpline number. (Contact details for Medic-Alert are on p. 96.) They should also inform all their friends, teachers and anyone with whom they are likely to be spending any time.

Living with anaphylaxis

Of course, it's frightening to discover that your child is suffering from any life-threatening condition. Fortunately, although it is something that everyone has to learn to live with, your child will be able to lead a normal life, with care. Treatment for anaphylactic shock is very effective and comes in the form of adrenaline injections, which are available on prescription for everyone – adults and children – believed to be at risk.

Adrenaline (sometimes known as Epinephrine) is available in measured doses in an 'Epipen' or 'Anapen'. It should normally be injected into the child's thigh as soon as a serious anaphylactic reaction is suspected. If there is no improvement within five to ten minutes a second dose should be given.

Using an Epipen is not difficult, but obviously you will feel much more confident about it if you have been shown how to do so. Ask if your GP or practice nurse, or the allergy nurse at the clinic, can show you what to do when an Epipen is prescribed for your child. The Anaphylaxis Campaign is planning to produce a training video – contact them for details of this.

An ambulance should always be called when anaphylactic shock is suspected. Even if the child responds to the Epipen injection she should be taken to hospital as soon as possible for observation and/or further treatment.

Of course, it is vitally important for everyone who looks after your child to know that she has a severe allergy and that she carries medication to treat it if it becomes necessary. However, part of the management of the condition consists of **allergen avoidance** – important for everyone with allergies, but especially so for a child whose allergies are life-threatening. You need to be as sure as you can possibly be that your child will not be exposed to the food or substance which upsets her.

This is much less difficult than it used to be, thanks to increased awareness of allergy among childminders, nurseries, schools, food manufacturers, supermarkets and the general public. Like the other campaigning groups, Allergy UK, the National Eczema Society and Asthma UK, the Anaphylaxis Campaign has worked hard with the Departments of Health and Education to ensure that schools have strategies in place to deal with children's special medical needs. Both Allergy UK and the Anaphylaxis Campaign have sample forms for parents to take into schools, nurseries or playgroups explaining exactly what the child's problem is, which substances he is allergic to, and what action is to be taken if the child does experience anaphylactic shock. It makes sense to have a written agreement between parents and schools/childminders so that everyone knows exactly what to do in the unlikely event of an emergency. Training in how to use emergency medication can often be provided by local GP surgeries, the school nurse department of the Local Education Authority or a paediatric nurse from the local hospital or allergy clinic. Carers should be certain they know

- which foods or products are likely to cause problems;
- what symptoms to look out for;
- where emergency medication is kept – normally in a safe place, easily accessible but away from other children;
- how and when medication should be used;
- how to contact the child's parents and GP and, if possible, another emergency contact such as a grandparent;
- when to call an ambulance.

It is often simpler for parents to provide a packed lunch, made with suitable ingredients, for an allergic child. All children should be told *not* to swap sandwiches with other children. Very little ones should, of course, be supervised while they are eating snacks and lunches. It is also important to remember that in some cases even the slightest contact with allergens may cause a reaction. Any spills should be wiped up straight away and hands washed. It's probably best for nursery schools and playgroups to avoid games and craft activities which use cardboard cereal packets that have contained cereals with nuts. Parents could provide 'safe' sweets or treats which can be shared on special occasions. It's also safer for class pets to be of the non-furry variety – stick insects, fish or giant snails are less likely to lead to an allergic reaction than hamsters or guinea-pigs. With older children, collages including nuts, seeds and pulses should be avoided. There's sometimes a question-mark over items like paints, glues, play-dough and other craft materials. Teachers should check with the child's parents and the product manufacturers and take all possible precautions.

The Anaphylaxis Campaign says that it's important to remember that severe reactions in young children are rare and that nurseries and schools do a fantastic job in keeping young children safe.

'We hear of half-a-dozen fatalities every year,' says David Reading.

However, there may be others which have been wrongly diagnosed or wrongly recorded. For example, there are approximately 1,400 asthma deaths a year; some of these may, in fact, be the result of anaphylactic shock. What we do know is that there are seven times as many hospital admissions as there were ten years ago, and the rate of hospital admissions has doubled in the last four years.

Letting go

It is worrying for the parents of a child with anaphylaxis to let anyone else care for their youngster. However, even severely allergic children need time and space to learn and play and enjoy the same range of childhood experiences as their non-allergic friends. An extremely useful publication from the Campaign is their booklet *Letting Go – Teaching an Allergic Child Responsibility*, which helps parents to strike the delicate balance between keeping a child safe and helping him to achieve independence and take control of his own environment. Tips include:

- staying calm when discussing the possibility of anaphylactic shock with the child and with others;
- boosting a child's self-esteem so that she has the confidence to say 'no' to anything from forbidden foods to drink and drugs;
- reading food labels together and identifying the allergens;
- encouraging her to remind her teachers or her friends' parents, or tell staff in restaurants, about what she can't eat. It is not rude or impolite to refuse, for instance, home-made cakes which might contain eggs, dairy or nuts.

'It's hard for me to feel really relaxed,' admits Gillian, whose 4-year-old daughter Megan is now at playgroup.

Meg is the first severely allergic child who has attended her playgroup. I have had to show them how to use her Epipen and explained that Megan risks anaphylactic shock if she comes into contact with eggs, nuts or milk. She is also allergic to pollen and animal fur.

Megan has been admitted to hospital three times already, the first after Gillian gave her egg at the age of ten months.

'She had always suffered a bit with eczema,' says her mum, 'but as soon as she ate the egg she came out in hives all over her body. Her lips swelled up, she started to choke and couldn't breathe, so we rushed her to hospital.'

Surprisingly, it took some time for Megan's doctors to diagnose an allergy, even though she ended up in intensive care on a ventilator the second time she went to hospital.

They didn't seem very allergy-aware, but eventually she was given allergy tests and treated with anti-histamines and, later, steroids. Since then we have avoided the foods we know are a problem but recently had a shock when she also reacted to some sunflower seeds in her morning toast. Half an hour later she went into anaphylactic shock and we had to use her Epipen, which worked brilliantly.

Shopping for children with anaphylaxis

Reading food labels becomes second nature when you are shopping for anyone with a food allergy (see Chapter 4). Food manufacturers and supermarkets are improving labelling all the time, but you need to be very sure that nothing your child eats puts him at risk. This makes food shopping complicated and time-consuming, even if you supply yourself with the supermarket and manufacturers' 'Free From' lists and only buy items you are sure about. Bear in mind that ingredients occasionally do change! A shopping survey by the Anaphylaxis Campaign in 2001 revealed that shoppers took 39 per cent longer when shopping for an allergic person than for someone with no allergies. Of 127 common food items, 71 carried a 'nut traces' warning and many were not suitable for those with nut allergies. Warnings were sometimes hard to find and difficult to read.

If you are at all unsure what a product contains, don't offer it to your allergic child.

Foods most likely to contain nuts or traces of nut products are:

- cakes, biscuits, pastries, ice-cream, desserts – even if they don't contain nuts they may have been made on the same factory production line or with the same utensils as similar products containing nuts;
- cereal bars and sweets;
- vegetarian products like veggie-burgers;
- salads and salad dressings;
- ready-made dishes in Chinese, Indian, Thai or Indonesian food ranges, for instance curries or satay sauce;
- marzipan and praline.

There is a question-mark over the safety of peanut oil – sometimes labelled 'groundnut oil'. Allergy UK have reported that some cosmetic creams contain 'arachis oil' – another name for peanut oil – but that this doesn't usually cause any problems. You may prefer to avoid such products as there are plenty of others on the market.

Just to confuse the issue, the peanut is actually a legume, and not a true nut. Other legumes include lentils, chickpeas, soya beans, black-eyed beans, butter beans, bean sprouts, even baked beans. Strangely enough, those with a peanut allergy are more likely to react to other nuts – 'tree nuts' like brazils or almonds – than they are to other legumes. The only way of finding out exactly which nuts affect your child is by proper allergy tests which your GP can arrange for him.

Eating out

Family meals out are a treat and there's no reason why children with allergies should miss out. It's easiest if you develop a relationship with local restaurants that you visit frequently. Ask the waiting staff, or the chef if possible, which items on the menu are guaranteed nut-, egg- or dairy-free. Remember that this could mean you have to avoid menu items fried in the same oil as those which do contain nuts or other allergens. As a general rule, plain food – grilled meat or fish with vegetables and salad without dressing – is a better bet. If the staff can't give guarantees of food safety, it's best to eat elsewhere. Chinese, Indian and other Asian restaurants tend to use a lot of nut oils in their cooking and it may be better to avoid this kind of food. As your child grows older, let *her* ask the questions.

'We advise families planning a meal out to phone the restaurant in advance and ask if they can provide an allergy-safe meal,' says David Reading.

When you're talking to the staff you need to be absolutely clear what your allergic child can and can't eat. On the whole, our members say that restaurants are much more aware and helpful than they were, say, ten years ago. Some are extremely good and offer an ingredients list or a booklet with details of how dishes are prepared. Others are anxious or afraid and say they can't help. We would like council environmental health officers – the 'food police', so-called – to make sure that restaurants are allergy aware.

'We went to the USA for our summer holiday because we thought at least we would be able to explain in English what Billy's problem was,' admits Lynn, whose 3-year-old son had an anaphylactic reaction to peanuts and is also allergic to eggs.

We found that the restaurants often had allergy information on their menus, but we also asked the managers which foods were safe to give him. Some panicked, but most were very helpful.

It is harder to eat out in Britain. We have a Turkish restaurant near us where the staff are very good. It's hard for Billy to have to refuse treats like chocolate. I always try to carry something in my bag that he *can* eat, so that he isn't too disappointed. Even at his age he knows he has to ask me if it's okay for him to eat something.

One of the hardest things is educating the people who spend time with him. One friend of mine is very good because her father has a dairy allergy so she is used to the idea of checking ingredients. She even made a special egg-free birthday cake which Billy could enjoy. Other people, though, sometimes forget to check.

How the law helps

The Food Standards Agency (FSA) is the government body in charge of things like food labelling. They say they are committed to funding research into food allergy and intolerance, and also to improving labelling.

At the moment there are laws about exactly what information must be given on food labels and these are constantly being updated. Currently, for instance, if an ingredient forms less than 25 per cent of a product (like sponge fingers in trifle) its ingredients don't have to be listed, though this may change in future. For a child who is at risk of anaphylaxis if he eats even a tiny amount of a particular ingredient, it's obviously important that *every* ingredient is listed. Food manufacturers are not legally obliged to use a 'may contain traces of nuts' label, though many do.

The FSA also says it is raising awareness of allergy among caterers, producing a *Be Allergy Aware* booklet and poster for catering companies and advising them to be sure their staff know what ingredients are being used. The British Retail Consortium and the Food and Drink Federation can also provide advice for catering establishments. At the moment, however, the onus seems to be on customers and parents to check the safety of all the food they buy.

When your teenager leaves home

By the time your teenager is old enough to leave home for college, to work away or take a 'gap year', she should be used to coping with her allergy and taking the responsibility for carrying her medication everywhere she goes. She may even have grown out of the problem. About 20 per cent of children do; the rest are affected for the rest of their lives. Colleges and universities are often very sympathetic towards students with special medical and dietary needs. If your child is going to live in catered accommodation, you will need to talk to the catering manager or supervisor about her requirements. If she is cooking for herself, make sure she gets plenty of practice in the family kitchen before she goes. The other vital thing is that she tells her new friends and flatmates about her allergies. Like her school friends and teachers, they should know the signs to look out for, and they should also know what to do in the event of an anaphylactic shock. David Reading of the Anaphylaxis Campaign says that it can be troublesome in teenagers, as once they fly the nest they don't have Mum and Dad around to remind them not to take risks and to carry their medication everywhere they go.

It's worth reminding teenagers that it is possible to have an allergic reaction to being kissed by someone who has just eaten peanuts, if you are especially sensitive to them! Also, when travelling, you can carry a translation card (available from Allergy UK) explaining the problem in a variety of languages.

Avoiding bee and wasp stings

The vast majority of cases of anaphylactic shock are caused by a reaction to food. Most of the members of the Anaphylaxis Campaign are allergic to food and it is a more complex problem, raising issues like the accuracy of food labelling and menu ingredients in restaurants. It's easier to avoid bees and wasps than it is to negotiate a minefield of food shopping. However, in Britain between two and nine people die every year after having a fatal reaction to bee or wasp stings. Those most at risk of developing anaphylaxis in these circumstances are children who are already known to be allergic to food, or who have allergic conditions like asthma or eczema.

If you have a severely allergic child, take special care when there are stinging insects around. If you are picnicking, avoid areas where there are bees or wasps, keep food covered before you eat it, stay away from dustbins which attract wasps, and watch what you eat – insects have been known to land on sandwiches or cakes and in drink cans! Keep children away from tree trunks and stumps, which sometimes house wasps' nests. Wipe sticky hands and faces with a damp flannel after eating.

Brightly coloured clothes attract insects, as do flowery prints and black. Encourage children to wear shoes when out of doors, and avoid highly perfumed products. Use insect repellent if you are outdoors a lot. Natural repellents are available if your child is allergic to chemical products (see p. 92 for details).

Teach your children not to panic if a bee or wasp lands on them. Instead, encourage them to keep calm and the insect will soon fly away. Bees, unlike wasps, are not naturally aggressive. Wasps can be aggressive, especially in the autumn when their supplies of food are running out. Check the car for bees and wasps before you get in.

6
Hay fever

Hay fever is poorly named, as it isn't caused by hay and it doesn't produce a fever! It's one of the most common allergic conditions, affecting somewhere between one in ten and one in five of the population in the UK. It's most common in children and young people, rare in the very young. One of the benefits of getting older is that hay fever becomes less severe. Like other allergic reactions, it appears to be becoming more common. It seems to have been virtually unknown before the early nineteenth century although Victorian sufferers were recommended a 'Carbolic Smoke Ball' to prevent and cure the symptoms! Many people with hay fever have other allergies as well. Boys are slightly more likely to have hay fever than girls and, surprisingly, it is more common in towns and cities than it is in the countryside.

What is hay fever?

A better – though more cumbersome – name for hay fever is 'seasonal allergic rhinitis'.

- **Seasonal** because it commonly affects people between spring and autumn. Hay fever is caused by pollen allergy, and those are the months when trees, grasses, weeds and moulds are producing pollen. If your child has the symptoms of rhinitis (an itchy, runny nose, sneezing, sore eyes, cough, tightness in the chest) all the year round, it's likely that he is allergic to something else – for example, house-dust mite or animal dander – instead of, or in addition to, pollen.
- **Allergic** means that like other allergies, hay fever is the immune system's response to normally harmless substances or allergens. The immune system perceives these as a threat and, in response, produces IgE antibodies. These stick to special cells in the body called 'mast cells' which release chemicals like histamines into the system, causing the well-known symptoms.
- **Rhinitis** means inflammation of the nose and nasal passages, although, as every sufferer knows, hay fever affects other organs

too. In addition to bouts of sneezing and a constantly runny nose, your child may have watery, itchy, reddened eyes, headaches, sleeplessness and general malaise.

Pollens and hay fever

If your child's hay-fever symptoms are most troublesome in spring, roughly between the end of February and late April, it's likely that tree pollen is responsible. Trees produce pollen shortly after their leaves develop. Species which cause problems include oak, elm, birch, ash, hazel and alder – in fact, most of Britain's commonest deciduous trees! Conifers also produce pollen but don't usually cause any problems as their pollen is non-allergenic.

The 'high season' for hay fever is, of course, the summer, roughly between mid-May and mid-August, when grass pollen is most widespread. Unfortunately for many teenagers, this often coincides with the examination season. If your child suffers badly from hay fever, you should make a point of explaining to his teachers what his difficulties are likely to be. For example, you could ask if he could have a seat as far away from open windows as possible to minimize his exposure to pollen.

Examination boards are generally sympathetic to students who have health problems, including hay fever. EdExcel, one of the biggest boards, say that allowances can be made for sufferers *as long as they are told in advance.*

'If an examination candidate suffers really badly from hay fever, the school or college should forward a letter from his doctor to us, explaining the problem,' says a spokesman.

In such cases we may be able to allow the candidate extra time to complete the papers, or a break during the exam if necessary.

It is also sometimes possible for a candidate's marks to be adjusted by up to 5 per cent if it is felt they could be affected by his hay fever. Or, if he is so badly affected he is unable to sit the exam, he could be awarded a mark based on the class average plus supporting evidence from his teachers or lecturers. We do try to help all students to have the best possible chance of reaching their potential. However, it is no use telling us about the candidate's hay fever after the results have come out, which does occasionally happen!

Grass pollen

There are literally hundreds of different kinds of grass, but relatively few are common enough, or produce enough pollen, to give the dreaded high pollen count. Types of grass include orchard grass, cocksfoot, rye grass, Yorkshire fog, meadow grass and timothy grass. How much pollen there is in the air and how it affects hay-fever sufferers will depend on the notoriously unpredictable British weather. Each type of grass sheds its pollen at a different time of day, often in the early morning, though some species flower for a second time in the late afternoon. On still days, pollen is deposited on the ground; with more of a wind it is carried away and deposited elsewhere later. On fine days, pollen is carried up into the atmosphere by warm air currents in the daytime. In the early evening, between 5 and 6 p.m., the pollen grains tend to fall in concentrated clouds, so in country areas this is often the time when the pollen count is at its highest. However, pollen clouds are blown into city areas later so the evening may be the worst time for city-dwelling hay-fever sufferers. Afternoon showers of rain can clear the air and mean a sneeze-free evening.

According to Dr William Bird, Medical Consultant to the Meteorological Office, thunderstorms can make hay-fever and asthma symptoms worse, because they fragment pollen grains. In July 2002 there were dramatic thunderstorms in Bedford, Norwich and Cambridge – followed by an increase in hospital admissions in patients with asthma symptoms.

Later in the year, in late August and September, hay-fever symptoms can be caused by mould spores. Moulds grow in warm weather in warm damp areas like compost heaps, or among rotting fruit. Some moulds grow on window frames where there has been condensation, others on ripening wheat and barley grain. All can cause hay-fever symptoms. Weeds like nettles, dock and plantain also flourish late in the season and weed pollen can be another cause of late-summer hay fever.

The pollen count

The 'pollen count' is part of every weather forecast these days, and has been since 1979. The UK Pollen Monitoring Network, based in Worcester, provides the figures. During the summer, the levels of pollen in the atmosphere are measured at 33 different places in the UK, ranging from Invergowrie in north-east Scotland to Newport, Isle of Wight, and from Belfast in the west to Ipswich in the east. The various sites are run by hospital allergy clinics, universities and colleges and environmental health offices. The information is sent to radio and TV stations and websites so that viewers and listeners can keep up to date. Pollen grains measure about one-twentieth of a millimetre across, so are invisible to the naked eye. Each grain contains several allergenic proteins. The pollen count actually measures the number of pollen grains in a cubic metre of air, and an average is taken over a 24-hour period.

Children who are especially sensitive to pollen might start to experience symptoms when the pollen count is as low as 10, though everyone's threshold is different. When it reaches 50, most sufferers will start to experience symptoms. In Britain, the count often rises to 200-plus in the summer. The highest pollen counts recorded were over 1,000, recorded in the Derby area in the 1970s.

Some parts of the UK seem to do better than others as far as pollen is concerned – perhaps due to the prevailing winds, perhaps as a result of other pollutants in the atmosphere, or relatively low rainfall. The Scottish Highlands, the Pennines, the East and West Ridings of Yorkshire and the Black Mountains of Wales have relatively low pollen counts, even in high summer, whereas land-locked areas of the Midlands, East Anglia and the South East of England have high pollen counts. Coastal areas tend to have lower pollen counts, especially west-facing coasts. Winds blowing from the west can deposit pollen on east coast beaches, which sometimes register higher than expected pollen counts.

Air pollution can make hay-fever symptoms worse as allergens attach themselves to pollution particles and get into the respiratory system. Breezy summer days can carry pollen from a 50-mile radius to affect city-dwellers as much as those living near to country meadows.

The start of the pollen season tends to vary around the country as well. People living in the South West can begin to be troubled by grass pollen allergies about five weeks earlier than those living in the north of Scotland. If we have a warm spring, with higher than average temperatures in March and April, plants grow more quickly and produce more pollen. Then the grass pollen season will start, and reach its peak, slightly earlier than normal.

We hear a lot about climate change and recent hot, dry summers at the beginning of the millennium have meant that hay-fever symptoms have started to appear earlier in the year. Birch pollens are starting to be troublesome in late March, whereas twenty years ago late April was a more common starting-point. The pollen season has also lasted longer. Warm weather with adequate rainfall can extend the grass pollen season into late August. Not only has the pollen count been high, but there have been, on average, more 'high pollen count' days in recent summers – which means more misery for hay-fever sufferers.

Avoidance strategies

Effective treatments for hay fever are available from your pharmacist or GP. Starting treatment a couple of weeks before the pollen season begins is often recommended. There is also quite a lot you can do to minimize the symptoms of hay fever, even when the pollen count is high. For example, you can

- make sure you are aware of the daily pollen forecast from radio or TV bulletins;
- on days when the pollen count is high, keep your child away from gardens and parks if possible, especially if the grass has just been cut;
- buy your child a pair of sunglasses, to protect his eyes from airborne pollen;
- make the most of cool, cloudy days for family outings;
- keep windows and doors closed, especially mid-morning and in the early evening;
- change your child's clothes when he comes indoors – pollen often becomes trapped in clothing;
- remember that a shower and a hair-wash can also help;
- choose a family car with air-conditioning or a pollen filter;
- smear a little Vaseline around the nostrils – it is soothing and can help trap pollen;
- try to keep your child away from smoky or polluted atmospheres;
- keep any pets out of the bedroom – pollen becomes trapped in their fur so bath your dog often or wipe him down with a wet-wipe;

- make sure you don't leave washing on the line when the pollen count is high;
- see Chapter 7 for more information about allergy-proofing your home.

Mum-of-five Janice is a hay-fever sufferer herself, as are her husband and four of their children.

'We live next to a park so we can't avoid pollens altogether,' she says.

We all take anti-histamines all summer, and wash our faces and hands when we come indoors. We have now got wooden floors in the living room and our bedrooms, and shutters or blinds at the windows rather than heavy drapes. We keep the windows closed at night, too, and I have a special Miele vacuum cleaner with a dust filter.

It's hard to say how much all this helps but at least the children aren't kept awake half the night coughing and sneezing. My daughter will be doing her GCSEs next year and I am worried about how it will affect her as the anti-histamines do make her feel groggy. We had a circular letter from her school saying they are thinking of changing over to a six-term year which would mean exams taking place in May, before the hay-fever season really starts.

Holidays

If you have a hay-fever sufferer in the family, you'll need to choose your holiday destination carefully. Coastal and mountain areas are a good choice, especially places with early seasons. For example, if you go to the Greek Islands or southern Turkey during the school holidays (July–August) the worst of the local pollen season – between mid-April and mid-June – will be over. The Portuguese Algarve has many west-facing coasts where pollen is less of a problem, and the west (Atlantic) coast of France also has generally low pollen counts. Grass pollen levels are high in May and June in Italy and Spain. The Balearics are also a good choice and, for later holidays, the Canary Islands. Alpine regions generally have low pollen counts. France, Italy and Scandinavia have efficient pollen monitoring systems, with information on local radio and in the newspapers. Tourist boards may be able to offer advice on this.

If you're planning to travel further afield, Egypt has a long pollen season so a winter trip will probably be best. Tropical areas like the Caribbean have lower levels of pollen between August and October. It's best to visit monsoon climates like India, Brazil or the Philippines just before the rainy season as most plants release their pollen once the monsoon is over. Areas with high humidity are more likely to have fungal growth, so if your child's hay fever seems to be mould-related you should bear this in mind.

Visitors to the USA should know that June is generally the worst month for grass pollen, although many states are affected between May and October. The plant which apparently causes most hay-fever symptoms in the USA is ragweed – known as 'sneezeweed'! – which releases its highly allergenic pollen between July and October in the eastern and mid-western states. Tree pollens can be a problem in Florida in the early months of the year. All American states issue 'pollen calendars' – ask your travel agent or local tourist boards for advice.

If you're planning to holiday in Britain, choose areas where the pollen count tends to be lower, like the Scottish Highlands or west coast resorts like Blackpool and Morecambe. Some of the companies producing hay-fever medication have helplines you can call for information about the pollen count.

Treating hay fever

Many hay-fever treatments are available over the counter. Ask your pharmacist's advice if you are not sure which is most suitable for your child, and consult your GP if they are not effective.

The most widely used drugs for hay-fever symptoms are **anti-histamines**. As their name suggests, their main action is to counter the effect of histamine, one of the chemicals released in the body when there is an allergic reaction. Anti-histamines relieve many of the most irritating symptoms including itching, sneezing, runny nose and streaming eyes. Brand names include Benadryl, Piriteze, Clarityn and Zirtek. Most are tablets but some are also available in the form of syrup (Clarityn, Piriton, Zirtek Allergy Solution) and are suitable for younger children. Boots and Lloyds Pharmacies make own-brand allergy relief tablets as well. **Always read the label and**

any instructions, as many of the most popular over-the-counter preparations are not recommended for children under 12.

Like most drugs, anti-histamines occasionally produce unwanted side-effects, the most common of which is drowsiness. Allergy UK's factsheet on hay fever points out that if your child needs to take anti-histamines on a regular basis, one of the newer brands which are non-sedating is a better option.

If your child's main symptom is a stuffy, blocked nose, or if anti-histamines don't seem to solve the problem, she may need additional medication in the form of eye or nose treatment. Decongestant sprays like Pollenase or Beconase should only be used on a short-term basis as long-term use can damage the delicate membranes in the nose, leading to dryness and discomfort. It's important to check with your pharmacist that anything you plan to use is suitable for your child's age group.

Boots have recently introduced Nasosal nasal drops which are suitable for adults and children over 2. The other drugs frequently used are **anti-inflammatories**, which come in two main types, **corticosteroids** and **sodium cromoglycate**. Although these work slightly differently from each other, the effect is to cut down on the number of inflammatory chemicals and the number of inflammatory cells in the eyes and nose. These medicines come in the form of nasal drops and sprays, aerosols, liquid sprays and eye drops.

If you know when your child's hay-fever symptoms are likely to begin to be a problem, it can help to begin on a course of anti-histamines plus eye or nose drops before the pollen season starts, to stop the worst symptoms developing. There can be occasional side-effects such as nosebleeds, but these medicines are effective and work well on the whole. If you're concerned about steroid use, it's important to remember that the amount of steroid in these preparations is very small and is unlikely to cause problems.

If over-the-counter treatments do not seem to be effective and/or your child is seriously allergic, your GP may be able to offer other forms of treatment. It is sometimes possible to be treated with steroid tablets or a long-lasting injection. This is called 'desensitiza-tion' or 'immunotherapy' and involves giving the patient a series of injections containing gradually increasing doses of the pollen allergen. Exactly how this works is not yet understood but, because there is a risk of serious allergic reaction, it must always be carried out under expert medical supervision.

Contact lenses

If your teenager wears contact lenses, ask your pharmacist's advice on which eye drops would be the most suitable, as some products dry up the eye's natural secretions and make contact lens wearing uncomfortable. Optometrist Iain Anderson of the Eyecare Trust says that hay fever affects the composition of the tear fluid in the eyes.

'Tear fluid is a mixture of oily secretions, water and mucus, and hay fever affects the balance of these,' he says. 'Sufferers may find their lenses get dirty more easily and their anti-histamines reduce tear flow. If a young person has a significant hay-fever problem then glasses may be a better bet.'

Complementary therapies

Some people prefer to use complementary therapies for hay fever, either because they are concerned about the side-effects of conventional drugs or because they prefer a 'natural' alternative. Allergy UK points out that a recent study in the *British Medical Journal* demonstrated that **homoeopathy** could be effective in treating rhinitis symptoms. Homoeopathy is said to work by stimulating the body's natural reaction to combat illness. A wide range of homoeopathic remedies is available over the counter in pharmacies and health-food stores, from companies like New Era, and also own-brand remedies from Boots.

Choosing the right homoeopathic medicine involves looking at a list of symptoms and personal characteristics and choosing the remedy which best fits the patient's symptom pattern. For example, you might choose Euphrasia for a child with very itchy, watery eyes, or Gelsemium for one who sneezed constantly. For a more detailed diagnosis it is best to consult a qualified homoeopath (contact details on p. 95).

Herbal medicine

Herbal medicine has been used for thousands of years to treat diseases, and many pharmaceutical drugs are derived from plant materials. Echinacea is a herb which is said to stimulate the immune system. Many herbal medicine companies produce their own hay-fever remedies like Potter's Antifect, which contains echinacea and garlic oil, or Medic Herb's Revitonil Echinacea, which contains a blend of soothing herbs. Research from Switzerland, published in the *British Medical Journal* in 2002, found that the herb butterbur was as effective as anti-histamines in treating hay fever. Pycnogenol, an extract of French maritime pine bark, has also been shown to be effective. Natural cosmetic company Weleda produces Rhinodoron Nasal Spray containing an aloe vera gel plus isotonic salt solution, said to soothe irritated nasal passages. For a detailed diagnosis it is best to consult a qualified medical herbalist.

Acupuncture

Acupuncture is a traditional Chinese form of treatment based on the idea that energy or 'chi' flows along meridians in the body, and that illness is the result of blockages in this energy. Acupuncture involves the insertion of very fine needles at specific points along these meridians, and is said to help some people with hay-fever symptoms, according to Allergy UK. To find the name of a qualified acupuncturist in your area contact the Acupuncture Council (contact details on p. 94).

Nasaleze

Another alternative to anti-histamines is a product called Nasaleze, an extract of cellulose powder which is said to enhance natural nasal mucus and 'filter out' the allergens which cause problems. The product performed well when tested by 102 hay-fever sufferers, who found it at least as effective as some of the over-the-counter anti-histamines. It is equally suitable for children and adults. Nasaleze is available from good health-food stores and independent pharmacies, or you can contact 01923 205704 for stockist details.

Professor Edzard Ernst, Britain's only professor of complementary medicine, who is based at the Peninsula Medical School, Exeter University, points out that there are, in fact, several properly conducted clinical studies of the effectiveness of 'alternative' hay-fever treatments. He describes the results for homoeopathy and some herbal medicines as 'promising' and those for acupuncture as' inconclusive'. Other suggestions, such as avoiding so-called 'mucus-producing' foods like dairy products and animal fat, do not seem to have scientific backing. However, every child can benefit from a healthy diet with plenty of fresh fruit and vegetables and as few over-refined, processed, sugary and fatty foods as possible!

7

Allergies and the environment

If your child suffers from any kind of allergy, you will want to reduce her exposure to environmental allergens as much as possible. Unfortunately, many children suffer from multiple allergies to a greater or lesser extent. Short of living in a completely sterile bubble, you can't avoid *everything* that makes her cough, or wheeze, or brings her out in hives or worsens her eczema. Nor would it be desirable if you could. The goal of allergy management is to enable children to lead normal or near-normal lives and take part in most of the same activities as their non-allergic friends.

For all but a small minority of allergy-prone children, this goal is an achievable one. Conventional drug treatments, like emollient creams for eczema and preventer and reliever inhalers for asthma, are very effective if used properly. There are different kinds, so if the one your child has been prescribed doesn't seem to be controlling the problem, go back to the GP or clinic and ask for something else. All allergy treatments should be regularly monitored, so that any medication can be adjusted if necessary. The use of some complementary therapies alongside conventional treatments for asthma sometimes seems to reduce a child's symptoms to the point where they need to use an inhaler less frequently, for example. However, it needs to be stressed that no reputable complementary therapist should suggest that a child stops using her medication.

Environmental factors affecting allergies

As doctors are not yet sure which factors in today's environment are to blame for the rise in allergies – it may also be a combination of factors – providing a healthy environment for your allergic child is always going to be a matter or trial and error. Country areas are not necessarily healthier than cities. Traffic pollution may exacerbate a tendency to asthma, but so may the chemicals routinely sprayed on Britain's farm crops. Prevailing winds mean that levels of pollution are not always higher in cities than they are in the countryside. Even if you have a choice, moving to the country might very well not solve your child's allergy problems. However, that doesn't mean there is nothing you can do to provide a healthier environment at home.

The only guaranteed way to discover exactly what triggers your child's problems is for him to be tested at a proper allergy clinic (for more information about allergy testing, see Chapter 8). Many parents also find this out through trial and error – if the child starts to wheeze on first contact with a cat, or when he goes into a flower-shop, for instance. Some allergens are easier to avoid than others, obviously. One of the most common, present in virtually every home and a frequent cause of allergic reactions, is the house-dust mite.

House-dust mites – the enemy within!

House-dust mites are tiny creatures, invisible to the naked eye, which live in their millions in even the cleanest of modern homes. They thrive on warmth and humidity, so modern, well-insulated, draught-proof houses with thick carpets, upholstered furniture, cosy duvets and lots of dust-gathering possessions are an ideal environment for them to grow and multiply. An ordinary mattress can contain up to 2 million dust-mite droppings and 10,000 dust-mites. According to Allergy UK, the average person loses 87 litres of sweat and 500 grammes of dead skin over the course of a year, so a bed is an ideal habitat for these little horrors. It has even been estimated that about 10 per cent of the weight of a pillow – more if it's an old one – is made up of dust-mite droppings, which cause allergic reactions in as many as 85 per cent of susceptible people! Although it would be very difficult to get rid of dust mites altogether, you can minimize the number of them in your home with some simple measures:

- Keep your home well ventilated by opening doors and windows.
- Vacuum carpets and floors frequently with a high filtration vacuum cleaner. Cleaners with HEPA (high efficiency particulate air) filters are quite widely available.
- Consider replacing your carpets and rugs with wooden or vinyl floors.
- Choose wipe-clean blinds for your windows rather than heavy fabric curtains which can trap dust mites.

- Consider replacing soft furnishings with leather or rattan furniture.
- Keep your home as cool as is comfortable. Think about putting on an extra sweater rather than turning the central heating up.
- Reduce humidity levels by not drying clothes indoors and by keeping bathroom and kitchen doors closed when you are cooking, washing or bathing. Relative humidity should be kept below 50 per cent. You can buy a hygrometer from your local hardware store to check the levels in your home.
- Use a damp cloth to dust, rather than a duster, to avoid spreading dust around.
- Consider investing in anti-allergy bedding. Washing bedding at 60°C will kill off dust mites, and you could look for special ranges such as the Fogarty 'Breath of Fresh Air' pillows, sheets and quilts, Relyon specially formulated mattresses, or Medivac covers which enclose your own mattress, duvet or pillow (contact details on p. 93).
- Reduce the number of cushions and other fabric accessories in your home. If your child has a lot of soft toys, wash them regularly at a high temperature or, alternatively, put them in the freezer for a time to kill the mites.
- Take a look at some of the anti-allergy sprays on the market, such as Total Hygiene DM 1 (stockist details on p. 93).
- Use one of the cleaning companies listed on p. 93 who specialize in allergy control.

Animal dander

Animal dander, which is a combination of flakes of animal skin and saliva, rather than actual fur, is another common cause of allergic reactions. If your child is allergic, the obvious answer is not to keep a pet, or at least not to keep a furry or feathered one. Perhaps your child could be persuaded to develop an interest in tropical fish or stick insects, or in sponsoring an exotic animal at a local zoo or animal rescue shelter? It is also important to make sure it is the pet which is causing the allergy, as having to think about re-homing a much-loved animal can be heartbreaking for the child and the whole family. The relationship between animals and allergies does not seem to be a straightforward one. Some studies have found that children brought up with pets are more likely to develop allergies, others that children who are in constant contact with animals – for instance on farms – are less likely to develop allergies. Theresa, whose 10-year-old son William has a severe peanut allergy, says that skin prick testing indicated that he is also allergic to cats.

'We have two cats at home, though, and William has never shown any reaction to them,' she says. 'His eyes do swell up if he goes near horses and we once had to take him to A&E because he could hardly see. Luckily, it didn't seem to affect his breathing and he showed no signs of anaphylactic shock.'

If you do decide to keep your pet, perhaps because your child has only a mild allergic reaction, you can help him by grooming the animal regularly. A product called Petal Cleanse, which claims to reduce the allergens in animal fur, can be used once a week, every week, to keep allergens down to an acceptable level. Petal Cleanse has been independently tested and can be used on both cats and dogs. It is made from mild detergents with the addition of aloe vera gel, rosemary, limeflower extracts and other natural products so it's safe for the animal as well, and has the backing of Allergy UK, Cats Protection, Battersea Dogs Home, the RSPCA and Greenpeace. (Stockist details on p. 92.) Simple Solution Allergy Relief Pet Wipes are also available from pet shops and pet superstores.

Eileen's 3-year-old grandson developed a severe allergy to her much-loved elderly cat. At first she thought re-homing the cat was the only option.

'I'd had him for 13 years since I found him in a dreadful state on the street,' she says.

One or two people even suggested he was so old I ought to have him put to sleep but I couldn't bear the idea. All the same, I hated not being able to see my grandson. He had had one severe asthma-type attack when he was rushed to hospital and given a nebulizer so my daughter wouldn't risk it a second time. I contacted cat rescue charities, and Cats Protection told me Petal Cleanse had worked with some of their cats whose owners had allergies. After about three treatments, my grandchildren came to stay again and Dean had no problems at all, only one puff from his inhaler all weekend!

Bathing a cat or dog is also said to reduce the amount of allergen in your home by 90 per cent, although if your cat hates being bathed this may not be an option! Some people find that the cat or dog breed makes a difference – some children react to long-haired but not short-haired breeds. Even if you do have to re-home your pet it may be some time before all traces of animal dander disappear from the house and you might find you have to clean carpets and upholstery several times, or even replace them, before the problem is eliminated.

Drug allergies

Some children react badly to antibiotics like penicillin and drugs in the same 'family', like amoxicillin, prescribed for bacterial infections. Reactions can range from fairly mild, for instance a skin rash, to swelling of the face and/or throat, to full-scale anaphylactic shock. **If your child has a bad reaction to a prescribed drug, obtain medical advice immediately.** Once you know your child is allergic, alternative antibiotics can be prescribed if they are needed. About 10 per cent of those allergic to penicillin-type drugs are also allergic to another class of antibiotics, the cephalosporins.

A report in the *British Medical Journal* in 2004 suggested that some asthma sufferers could be at risk of a severe allergic reaction to aspirin. Aspirin is no longer recommended as a treatment for children under 12, but if you have an asthmatic teenager it's worth bearing this in mind and choosing an alternative painkiller like paracetamol if necessary.

Chemicals in the home

In a special report in the *Guardian* newspaper in May 2004, a toxico-pathologist at Liverpool University was quoted as saying that from the moment they are conceived, today's children are exposed to 'a soup of chemicals, most of which would not have existed when our grandparents were in the womb'. Certainly, a glance at the ingredients contained in such everyday products as shampoo or floor cleaner can seem rather frightening. Although the exact relationship between the use of household chemicals and the rising incidence of allergies has not yet been established, many parents find that using some of the alternative, allergy-friendly products now available does help. Some carry the Allergy UK logo so you could look out for this. However, there is no absolute guarantee that making a lot of expensive changes to your child's home environment will benefit him. Unfortunately, it's not that easy!

Elizabeth, whose 10-year-old son David has eczema and is also allergic to penicillin, says she has tried all kinds of 'alternative' products with very mixed results.

'David's skin does flare up from time to time, especially in hot weather, and if he is stressed,' she explains.

Even small children can get stressed, especially if they are self-conscious about their skin! I wasn't happy about using steroid creams so I was always looking for alternatives. I tried different eco-friendly washing powders, and I tried washing David's clothes separately, but that didn't help. I did get fed up with spending money on things that didn't work. We changed our carpets for wooden floors, but I'm not sure how much difference that made. I avoided soap and tried cutting dairy and citrus fruit out of David's diet, to no avail. One thing that did make a noticeable difference was the Total Hygiene DM 1 spray which I used to spray his bedding. I've been using it for four months now and it has helped.

The effect of household products and toiletries on allergies is still being debated. Many allergy specialists say there is no proven link between the use of chemicals in the home and the rise in the number of children with allergies, and that the use of 'eco-friendly' products is pretty much a waste of money. Manufacturers point out that all household chemicals are thoroughly tested before they are permitted to go on the market. Even if some of the ingredients are proven to be harmful when, for instance, large quantities are injected into laboratory rats, the amount used in the products we buy is so small that it is unlikely to have any adverse effects. It is also perfectly possible to have an allergic reaction to something which is completely 'natural' – nettle rash being an obvious example. There are plenty of natural poisons!

However, environmental campaigners like Friends of the Earth and the Women's Environmental Network say that no studies have been done into the build-up of combinations of these chemicals in the human body over years and years. They say that it could be better to 'play safe' and minimize the number of products you use on your children's skin – and in your home.

The Women's Environmental Network (WEN) has been campaigning for some time in favour of the use of 'real nappies' rather than disposables. They say that not only are real nappies more environmentally friendly and cheaper to use, but they are healthier for babies' sensitive skin and less likely to cause allergic reactions. Slimline modern disposables contain chemicals, the long-term effects of which are not yet known. Real nappies, by contrast, can be made of 100 per cent organic cotton, unbleached and pesticide-free. Raw silk nappy-liners are also available. UK Nappy Line (contact details on p. 88) can give you information. The WEN website (contact details on p. 96) has up-to-date lists of acceptable baby products.

Cosmetics and toiletries

In response to consumer demand for purer, more 'natural' products, companies have started to produce certified organic and irritant-free skincare and other toiletries. Boots and other mainstream companies produce hypo-allergenic ranges which suit some skins. Charlotte Vohtz, founder of the Green People organic skin- and homecare company, began by producing skincare products suitable for her 2-year-old daughter who suffered from eczema and skin allergies. Margaret Weeds, who founded the Essential Care sensitive skincare company, is an aromatherapist and herbalist who began making products to treat her own children's skin problems twenty years ago.

'Parents of allergic children need to know exactly what is in the products they are buying,' she comments.

Some GPs only seem able to suggest hydrocortisone creams or emollients containing parabens, which people with eczema often can't tolerate. Our flagship products include Rescue Lotion, which is a 100 per cent concentration of aloe vera, and our Ultra Rich emollient made from cold-pressed plant oils and waxes plus St John's Wort, which is very effective against skin bacteria.

Other names to look out for are Barefoot Botanicals, Neal's Yard Remedies, Organic Blue and Little Me, the last-named being a specially formulated baby brand, again produced by a mother who couldn't find anything suitable for her own child. The Organic Pharmacy in London's King's Road sells a variety of own-brand and organic toiletries, including some for babies and children. (Contact details for these products on p. 92.)

Household chemicals

Just as some children with sensitivities react to toiletries, some of the ingredients in household cleaners can cause allergic reactions. Allergy-free products are available – Allergy UK has details and they are also widely advertised in their magazine, so you should be able to find products your child can tolerate. There are even companies making ranges of 'natural' paints and varnishes. (Addresses on p. 93.)

Many parents of allergic children choose to replace carpets and rugs with wooden floors. The Women's Environmental Network and Action Against Allergy (contact details on p. 86) set up the Healthy Flooring Network in 2000, with the aim of raising awareness of the links between fitted carpets, PVC flooring and health, particularly asthma and other allergic conditions. They point out that carpets harbour dust which leads to a build-up of dust-mite allergen, airborne particles and animal dander. Carpets may also contain the residues of chemicals used in their manufacture or treatment. Small children spend a lot of time on the floor and so come into more frequent contact with these possible allergens. The Swedish health authorities, concerned at the rise in the numbers of children with allergies, made a recommendation as long ago as 1989 that fitted carpets should not be used in schools, nurseries, offices and other public buildings. WEN can send interested parents a list of alternative flooring suppliers.

One of the best and simplest ways of improving your child's home environment is, of course, to make sure he lives in a non-smoking house. Exposure to tobacco smoke can trigger asthma attacks in susceptible children and 'passive smoking' is known to cause problems. Babies born to smokers are more likely to suffer from respiratory difficulties, so if you are planning a family, it's time to give up. Contact Quitline (details on p. 96) for information about the best ways to do this.

Air purifiers are also widely advertised in the Allergy UK magazine.

Latex allergy

This is another allergy which seems to be on the increase and which can affect children as well as adults, as mum-of-five Janice discovered.

'My youngest son Robbie has multiple food allergies, asthma and hay fever,' she says.

We also found out he was allergic to latex when we took him for his first haircut and the hairdresser put a rubber cape around his shoulders. His neck swelled up immediately, which was very alarming.

It affects all kinds of things, like children's parties where there are balloons, and I even have to be careful buying things like socks and underwear. I have discovered that Marks and Spencer socks and pants don't have latex in the elastic. Robbie is also very sporty and finding suitable items like swimming goggles and sports equipment has been very difficult. Latex can be used in school equipment like rubbers, glue, paints and crayons so I do a 'latex walk' around his new classroom every year!

There is a Latex Allergy Support Group – contact details on p. 94. They say that latex can crop up in unlikely places and recommend that you contact them for information about this. 'Latex' refers to natural rubber latex from the *Hevea brasiliensis* tree, grown in Malaysia and Thailand. Apparently, stretchy rubber products like rubber gloves and rubber bands are more likely to cause a reaction than harder ones like car tyres. If your child has a latex allergy it's important that any healthcare professionals with whom he comes into contact, like your GP, practice nurse or dentist, are aware of it so that they don't wear rubber gloves when examining him.

It is also possible that a child with latex allergy might react to fruits and vegetables like banana, kiwi, avocado, tomato or potato, which contain similar proteins.

Multiple allergies

As Janice has found, having a child or children with multiple and/or severe allergies can affect your family life in ways that you might not anticipate.

'We are used to reading food labels in our family,' she says.

When Robbie was small he used to ride in the trolley at the supermarket until I realized that when I pushed him past the fresh fish counter or the bakery he would begin to cough or start to itch. It's not just that he can't eat fish, we can't have fish in the house. One of the other children spilled some milk at breakfast one morning and it splashed on to Robbie's clothes. Although I undressed him and popped him under the shower straight away, he still came out in awful red blotches.

It can be quite difficult socially. As the mother of a severely allergic child you need to develop a thick skin and find the strength to stick up for your child, even when it doesn't come naturally to you. For example, Robbie has a severe nut allergy so when he was about to start nursery school I asked the staff if the nursery could become a nut-free zone. I got into all sorts of heated debates with other parents whose children wouldn't eat anything except peanut butter in their sandwiches!

My mother-in-law finds it hard, too. Like all grans she loves to buy the children treats and I'm sure she thinks I am just being neurotic or over-protective when I tell her there are lots of things they just can't eat.

Older generations, who brought their children up not to be 'faddy' and to eat everything that was put in front of them, may find it hard to adjust to visiting grandchildren who really can't eat some kinds of food. There may also be issues with friends and family who are unwilling to re-home pets because a child has an allergy. Tact and understanding on all sides are required here.

Some grandparents are too nervous to enjoy the company of allergic grandchildren in case they go into anaphylactic shock, as Becky, mother of severely allergic 5-year-old Ryan, explains.

'Mum panicked completely when Ryan was diagnosed,' she says.

Even now I have explained to her exactly what he can and can't eat and that he might also react to house-dust mites, cats, dogs and has sensitive skin that blisters in rain or bright sunshine, she is still really nervous with him. On the whole, it's better if friends and relations visit us, then they can see how we manage Ryan's allergies.

71

As far as creating an allergen-free home is concerned, I just do what I can. We have wooden floors, window blinds, no pets and very few soft toys. I damp-dust and try to use eco-friendly cleaning products.

We have strict protocols around eating in our house. Ryan has his own food cupboard and I cook his meals separately, using his own pans and serving them on his own plate. We wash our hands after eating, as well as before, and we only ever eat in the kitchen and dining-room, never elsewhere in the house.

Brothers and sisters of severely allergic children can also get a rough deal, as so much attention is necessarily given to the child with the allergy. Ryan has a 7-year-old brother who has no allergy problems at all.

'We have done our best to ensure that Brendan knows he is special too,' Becky comments.

He is very bright and positive and loves looking after his brother and making him laugh. Ryan has to go to London for tests every six months and Brendan comes with us to keep his brother company. Both boys get a treat afterwards. Brendan knows almost as much about what Ryan can and can't eat as I do and will advise his gran from time to time. His dad and I sometimes take him out for meals without his brother, so that he never gets the feeling he is being left out.

Holidays

Most families with allergic children find that self-catering holidays are their best bet as they can take suitable food from home and prepare it in familiar ways. If you use dust-mite-proof sheets on the child's bed at home, take them with you. Occasionally, flying can be a problem, especially since September 11th, 2001, as airlines are now so security-conscious that they may be unwilling even to let you take your child's Epipen in your hand luggage. Check what the airline's policy is before you go. You may need to provide yourself with a doctor's note to the effect that this is an essential piece of medical equipment which should be available at all times.

Another possible difficulty on flights is that peanuts are often served with drinks, and if your child is severely allergic, even inhaling peanut-scented air might cause a reaction. Again, check with the airline. With the rising number of allergies, some have decided not to serve peanuts.

If you're worried about language problems, Allergy UK has produced Allergy Alert cards in English and foreign languages explaining your allergies so that you can order in restaurants or explain what substances cause problems for you. Contact Allergy UK for details.

Many of the companies which produce 'natural' cosmetics and toiletries include things like sunscreens and mosquito repellent so you don't need to use a product that irritates your child's sensitive skin. Look for names like Dr Hauschka, Green People, Weleda and Neal's Yard Remedies.

Asthma UK runs PEAK holidays which are adventure holidays especially for youngsters with asthma, eczema and other allergic conditions, including food allergies. Children between 6 and 12, and young people between 12 and 17, are carefully supervised by trained volunteers and health professionals with access to emergency treatment nearby if required. As well as normal holiday experiences like swimming, games and visits to theme parks, there are educational activities aimed at helping the kids to manage their condition. PEAK holidays give children the opportunity to meet others with similar conditions and enjoy independent living in a safe environment. Contact Asthma UK for details.

8

Allergy testing

In order to work out the most effective form of treatment for your child's allergies, and to avoid the substances which cause an allergic reaction as far as possible, it's important that he is correctly diagnosed. In the Royal College of Physicians' 2003 report *Allergy – the Unmet Need* it was pointed out that Britain's allergy care lags behind that of other countries. Put simply, we have far too few allergy specialists, particularly paediatric allergy specialists (those experienced in the diagnosis and care of children with allergic diseases).

A lot of day-to-day allergy care is provided by GPs, many of whom have had no clinical training in the subject. Many of the calls to the helplines run by Allergy UK and the Anaphylaxis Campaign come from worried parents who report that there is no allergy clinic in their area and that their GP is unable to help. Most of the specialist clinics in the UK are in London and the South East; provision in the rest of the country is described as 'poor'. Again according to the RCP, in 2003 there were only six major centres staffed by consultant allergists offering a full-time service, with a further nine offering a part-time service. There are only 'a handful' of paediatric allergy specialists, compared to 96 in Sweden and 2,000 in Japan. Perhaps because of this, there are many private clinics offering 'allergy testing' of all types, varying from iridology (examination of the eyes) to hair analysis. Many of these 'alternative' kinds of allergy testing remain either unproven or unreliable, and are not recommended by the medical profession or by organizations like Allergy UK.

Even if it is obvious that your child has an allergy of some kind, it's important to see your GP or practice nurse to get a proper diagnosis. Your GP will need to know

- if there is a family history of any kind of allergy (asthma, eczema, hay fever, food allergies);
- whether the problem occurs at a particular time of the day, or year, and how often;
- how the child is affected – wheezing, coughing, swelling, itching, skin rash;

- how severe the symptoms are;
- if there is anything which makes the problem worse/better.

Your answers to these questions will help your doctor to decide on the most appropriate course of action, which will probably include allergy tests.

Skin prick testing

This is the most common kind of allergy test currently in use as it is relatively simple, quick and inexpensive. Skin prick testing can be done in a GP surgery or hospital clinic by specially trained nurses or doctors. It is designed to measure the IgE antibodies produced in response to particular allergens which can be anything from food (wheat, dairy, strawberries, etc.) to animal dander, pollens, house-dust mites, latex and certain drugs. Skin prick testing can be used on children of any age although it is not always reliable when used on small babies. Depending on the child's history of allergic reactions, a very few allergens – perhaps three or four – may be tested at one time, or as many as 25.

Skin prick testing is usually carried out on the child's inner forearm, although if she has bad eczema in that area it can be done on the back. A drop of a commercially produced allergen is placed on the skin, which is then pricked using the tip of a lancet. The test can be uncomfortable, but should not be painful. A marker pen is used to identify each individual allergen.

The results of a skin prick test can be seen within about 15 minutes. If the child has a 'positive reaction' the skin will soon become itchy and a raised weal, looking like a nettle sting, appears. The size of the weal varies from about 3 to 5 mm across.

Normally, in order to be sure of the diagnosis, both positive and negative controls are included among the skin prick tests. The negative control is a harmless solution of salt water, to which no reaction is expected. If your child reacts to this it means that her skin is exceptionally sensitive and special care is needed with her diagnosis. The positive control is a solution of histamine, to which everyone should react. If your child doesn't, it could be because she is on some kind of medication, perhaps an anti-histamine or even cough medicine. You should always tell the medical staff if your child is taking anything before she has a skin prick test.

Skin prick testing is very safe as the amount of allergen used is tiny, though if your child has suffered an anaphylactic reaction in the past it may not be appropriate.

Lynn's toddler son Billy had a bad reaction to peanut-butter cookies and was rushed to his local paediatric A&E department.

'By the time we saw a doctor his symptoms – a streaming nose, swollen lips and tongue and what looked like nettle-rash – had subsided,' says Lynn.

> He was prescribed an anti-histamine and steroids, but nothing was said about anaphylaxis, about avoiding possible triggers, or about treatment with an Epipen.
>
> My GP did later give us an Epipen and we were referred to the private Portland Hospital after two and a half months, where Billy was given skin prick tests. We found them rather traumatic as he had to sit still while the drops were put on his hand, and of course 2-year-olds don't keep still easily! He reacted positively to peanut, egg and dairy. We questioned the 'dairy' diagnosis as he loves milk, cheese and yogurt. In the end we changed to soya products. However, the next time he was tested he came up negative for dairy products and he seems able to tolerate them now.

Regular testing is important as children's allergic responses do seem to change with time. Five-year-old Ryan, who has multiple allergies, goes for skin prick testing every six months which means that his mum Becky can now vary his diet.

'His first skin prick tests came up positive for dairy, wheat, soya and cheese, and as I breast-fed him until he was $2\frac{1}{2}$ we both ate a very restricted diet,' she says.

> It was eighteen months before we were referred to a consultant at St Mary's in London, who tested him again. He reacted positively to a huge number of foods – lentils, garlic, peas, melon, peanuts, seeds, bananas and cucumber – as well as having a low-level allergic reaction to cats, dogs and house-dust mites. Later tests showed he had grown out of the reaction to wheat which means that I can now bake my own bread for him.

Blood tests

Sometimes known as RAST tests, these are tests which measure the amount of IgE circulating in the blood in response to a suspected allergen. RAST, in case you're wondering, stands for RadioAllergo-Sorbant test. A small sample of blood is taken, usually from a vein in the child's arm, using a fine needle and a small syringe. The blood sample is sent away to a hospital laboratory and results are available in a week or two. The tests can be carried out by your GP or practice nurse or in a hospital clinic.

Blood tests may be carried out when skin prick testing is thought to carry a high risk of anaphylactic shock. They are appropriate for children with very severe eczema, and are also used if a particularly rare allergy is suspected. Blood testing is very safe, though occasionally 'false negative' results occur.

Results are given on a scale of 0 (negative) to 6 (extremely high).

Patch tests

Patch testing is used when a child has eczema and is often carried out in dermatology departments. Allergens are mixed with a substance such as Vaseline and spread on to special non-allergenic discs which are placed on the skin and left for 48 hours, during which time the skin must be kept dry.

After this time, the patches are removed and the skin is examined for any redness or swelling. Interpreting the results can be a complex business and is best done by an experienced dermatologist, taking the child's medical history into account. Healthy people with no allergies sometimes react unexpectedly to patch testing. Like all such tests, it is not infallible.

Challenge tests

These involve exposing the child to the allergen which is thought to cause the problem, at first in minute and then in gradually increasing doses. 'Food challenge tests' involve giving the child a very small amount of the food to which he may be allergic. Five-year-old Ryan, who has multiple allergies, goes to hospital for challenge tests once a year.

'He has to take the tests in hospital with an intensive-care unit standing by in case of severe reactions,' says mum Becky. 'They usually try a skin prick first, then wait 20 minutes, then put a tiny bit on Ryan's lip and if that's okay they'll try a tiny bit more and a bit more after that.'

In order to discover exactly which foods cause the problems, different foods may be fed individually to the child in the form of capsules, so that he doesn't know what he is trying. In some tests, neither the child nor the doctor knows which food is being given, and someone else keeps the records – this is known as a double-blind food challenge. For children with severe or complex multiple allergies it is important to know which foods can and cannot be tolerated. Then an appropriate 'exclusion diet' can be worked out with the help of a paediatric dietician who can help parents make sure their child eats a balanced and nutritious diet, in spite of his allergies. (For more information on food allergy see Chapter 4.)

Other tests

Allergy testing is continually being refined and improved. At the same time, many complementary and alternative health clinics offer a range of tests which claim to identify and diagnose allergies. Most of these have not been submitted to the same rigorous scientific studies as more conventional testing methods. Those which have, have often been found to be of 'no proven value'. Among the most frequently offered tests are the following:

- The Vega test measures small changes in the electrical resistance of the skin in response to test substances. According to an article in the *British Medical Journal* in 2001, which was later quoted in the Royal College of Physicians' (RCP) allergy report, this sort of testing 'cannot be recommended for the diagnosis of environmental allergies'.
- In hair analysis, you send a hair sample off to a private laboratory to be tested, based on the idea that a person's state of health can be diagnosed from the condition of their hair. The RCP report says that the vitamin/mineral content of hair can affected by age, gender and geographical location.
- In the NuTron test, a blood sample is mixed with over 90 'pure food solutions' in a lab and then tested for neutrophils, a type of

white blood cell which seems to be involved in food intolerance. The RCP says there is no research evidence to support the efficacy of this kind of testing.

- Iridology diagnoses a patient's state of health by studying the pigment flecks on the iris of the eye. The RCP has found no valid evidence for this.
- Applied kinesiology measures muscle strength before and after exposure to a suspected allergen. Again, there is no independent evidence that this is effective.
- In leuko-cytotoxic testing, a drop of blood, plus food extract, is examined for changes to the white blood cells which are supposed to indicate an allergy. There is no independent evidence that this is effective.
- The Auricular Cardiac Reflex Method measures the strongest pulse at the wrist. The RCP report says this is unproven and that results are likely to be affected by the patient's state of anxiety while being tested.

If you are considering a non-standard type of allergy testing, always ask the clinic or practitioner for evidence that it has been subjected to clinical trials and written up in one, or more, peer-reviewed reputable scientific journal.

The YorkTest

Allergy UK has recently begun to recommend the 'YorkTest', a blood test for food intolerance, which can be done by post and also through Lloyds and Moss Pharmacy outlets. A double-blind, randomized controlled clinical trial of 150 subjects with Irritable Bowel Syndrome found that this test, which claims to identify food intolerances and then place subjects on an appropriate diet, could be effective. Clinical trials are now taking place to see whether the YorkTest is equally useful in treating patients with eczema and migraine. The YorkTest can be used for children from about $2\frac{1}{2}$ years old, but is not designed to identify classical allergies. (For details of how to find out more about the YorkTest, see p. 96.)

From time to time, allergy screening is offered on a 'walk-in' basis in supermarkets and pharmacies. This usually involves blood tests which, although they may be accurate, really need to be interpreted by a doctor so that a proper diagnosis can be made and treatment prescribed. The same applies to home testing kits. If you want to be sure your child's allergies are correctly diagnosed and that he is receiving appropriate treatment, including a healthy diet, it's better to press for a referral to an allergy specialist.

9

What about the future?

In her Foreword to the 2003 report *Allergy – the Unmet Need*, Professor Carol Black, the President of the Royal College of Physicians, says that at present there are far too few specialist allergists to meet the needs of the population. What the country needs, the report says, is more consultants, a network of accessible allergy centres around the country, and much improved and wider training of those who care for patients. 'These proposals,' the report concludes, 'require urgent action.' Since the report came out, with pressure from the different allergy charities and other interested parties in the medical profession, the Parliamentary Health Committee has established an enquiry into clinical allergy services for the UK.

Medical professionals involved in allergy care agree that more resources are needed so that all children have access to specialist allergy care if they need it. So do the parents of allergic children. Most of them have nothing but praise for the care their children receive when they do manage to see a specialist, but there are at present not nearly enough specialists to go round.

'I had to wait two months before my son was given food allergy tests, and I have since heard of families waiting for six months or more,' says one mother. 'GPs need to know more about allergies, too. I still hear of GPs who don't believe a child can be allergic to cow's milk.'

The Department of Health claims that the government's extra investment in the NHS will improve allergy services and points out that the Medical Research Council spent £3 million on asthma research in 2001–2, including research into the relationship between asthma and other allergies.

Muriel Simmonds, Chief Executive of Allergy UK, says that government funding should be spent on treatment centres as well as research.

'We have calculated that it would only cost £10 million to set up an allergy service,' she says. 'That's nothing when you think how much is already being spent on treating allergy-related conditions, and it might prevent children being on medication for the rest of their lives.'

Research into allergies is ongoing both in this country and abroad. Early in 2004 the Global Action on Allergy and Asthma European Network was launched. This is a five-year research programme, co-ordinated by Paul von Cauwenberge, Dean of the Medical Faculty at the University of Ghent in Belgium, and involving 25 universities and research institutes. More than £9 million of European Commission funding has been put into this project, which is concentrating on the different aspects of modern life which are said to have influenced the increase in allergies over the past ten or twenty years. Researchers are hoping that they will find the answers to the questions which have puzzled doctors for so long – the link between what we eat and where and how we live and bring up our families, and the allergic conditions that develop in so many of our children. Professor von Cauwenberge is hoping that better and simpler diagnostic tests and better treatments will emerge as a result of this research.

Professor John O. Warner, Professor of Child Health at South-ampton General Hospital, who is one of the country's leading experts on childhood allergies, says that, at the moment, researchers are looking at

- genetics and the part inheritance plays in the development of allergies;
- the 'Hygiene Hypothesis' – are our modern homes really too clean?
- early allergen avoidance and high-dose allergen exposure in infancy;
- nutritional influences on the allergic immune response;
- early drug treatments;
- new forms of immune modulation.

It is possible that, in the future, babies in the womb as well as infants and toddlers may be treated with allergens to build up their natural defences. DNA vaccines are also at an early stage of research.

Professor Warner believes that research should be focused on *prevention* of allergies, so that the mechanisms by which allergies develop in the first place can be better understood. At present, there is no way of knowing which allergies a child who is born into an atopic family will develop, or when. There are cases of brothers and sisters, even of identical twins, where one child suffers from a range of allergies and the other is allergy-free – but no one knows why. Even the experts still have a lot to learn.

Preventing asthma

Asthma UK, which funds research into the prevention and treatment of asthma in both children and adults, has published its strategy for future research after consulting 60 of the UK's leading asthma scientists. The single most urgent priority was identified as primary prevention of the development of asthma in children.

'Investigating what causes asthma to develop in children will help us to understand what early actions could lead to the prevention of asthma,' they say.

Asthma UK is also working on better diagnosis and assessment of asthma, treating those with very severe symptoms, and looking at alternative non-drug approaches to managing the condition as well as the best ways to manage asthma emergencies.

Improving diets for pregnant women

One of the most promising areas of research has involved looking at the effect of pregnant women's diets on the development of allergic diseases in their babies. Professor Warner has suggested that as many as 75 per cent of asthma cases could be prevented if mums-to-be were encouraged to eat a more appropriate diet in the final three months of pregnancy. Scientists have suggested that eating too many saturated fats and too little fruit, vegetables and Vitamin E during pregnancy can increase the risk of babies developing allergies.

Immunotherapy

Paediatric allergist Dr Jonathan Hourihane says that more and better training in allergy for primary care staff including GPs and practice nurses would help. 'At the moment, waiting times to see a specialist allergist are too long even after a child has suffered an anaphylactic reaction,' he says. 'There are only about half-a-dozen units like mine in the country, where we need one or two in every region.'

Dr Hourihane would also like to see the re-introduction of 'immunotherapy' as a treatment for allergies. This treatment involves injecting a tiny amount of the protein derived from a particular allergen under the skin of the patient and then giving them increased doses, a little at a time, to increase their tolerance. Immunotherapy was used in Britain in the 1980s, but unfortunately a few patients died. The field has moved on since then and immunotherapy is available as a treatment elsewhere in the world. It doesn't work for all allergies, but controlled studies have found that it can be effective in treating hay fever, mild allergic asthma, and allergy to bee and wasp stings. Some studies also suggest it works for cat dander and house-dust mite allergies, but not, as far as is known, for eczema or food sensitivity. Because it involves exposing patients to substances to which they are known to be allergic, immunotherapy can only be recommended for use by experienced allergists in specialist allergy centres. Dr Hourihane is currently studying 'oral immunotherapy', for which no injections are necessary, and says that if safety trials are successful this may be introduced in Britain in the next two or three years. It appears that children's responses to oral immunotherapy are long-lasting, so this could be a promising method of treating some forms of allergy in the future.

Other research projects worldwide seem to be finding clues to the causes of the allergy epidemic, and possible future treatments, although research is at an early stage. For example, researchers in Japan have identified a compound in green tea which, in laboratory tests, seemed to block the production of histamine and IgE.

Another research project, at the University of Turku in Finland, examined the 'Hygiene Hypothesis' and tried to establish whether exposure to so-called 'friendly' bacteria during infancy could help to establish the body's natural defences. A group of 132 pregnant women whose babies had been identified as at risk of developing allergic disease, were given either supplements containing Lactobacillus GG, or a placebo (dummy) pill, during the last weeks of their pregnancy and the first months of their babies' lives. The probiotic supplements were found to halve the risk of the babies developing eczema.

Dr Simon Murch of London's Royal Free Hospital was quoted as saying that 'If this is confirmed in other studies and is applicable to other allergic diseases, probiotics would represent an important therapeutic advance.'

As yet, the reason why these 'friendly bacteria' should have an effect on the development of allergies is not known. The National Eczema Society says that there are current studies trying to establish whether probiotics can help children and adults who already have eczema, and that more research is needed before they can confirm that probiotics have a role to play in preventing the disease, but that early signs are hopeful.

As it is already known that genetics plays a part in the development of allergic diseases, a British team under Professor Cookson in Oxford are studying the molecular genetics of eczema. They have already discovered that the genes containing susceptibility to asthma and those for eczema are quite different – it had previously been thought that they were the same.

New treatments

New treatments for allergic conditions are continually being introduced. These include Tacrolimus ointment and Pimecrolimus cream – otherwise known as Protopic and Elidel – which are **immunomodulators**. As their name suggests, these are non-steroid drugs which are able to alter the immune system, and are the first effective alternative treatments for eczema since topical steroids were introduced. Pimecrolimus is licensed for use in children over 2 and is suitable for treating mild to moderate eczema. Tacrolimus comes in two strengths and is licensed for use in children over 2 with moderate to severe eczema who have not responded to other treatments. However, as with all new drugs, the long-term effects are not yet known. Exactly which treatment suits your child best is something you should discuss with your GP and dermatologist.

10
Further help

Allergy is a complex subject and there are many organizations out there offering help and support to those affected. The major support groups have a dual role – pressing for more medical and social help, financing research projects and raising awareness among the medical profession and general public on the one hand, and offering support to affected families on the other. They produce a range of useful literature, send out regular newsletters with updates on the latest products and research findings, and some offer local support. Contact details are:

Action Against Allergy
PO Box 278
Twickenham TW1 4QQ
Website: www.actionagainstallergy.co.uk
Email: aaa@actionagainstallergy.freeserve.co.uk
AAA is a small membership organization which is a good source of information for those affected by allergies. They offer practical help, plus leaflets on allergy-related subjects including special diets and hotels suitable for those with allergies. They also have a database of local allergy specialists. They can't deal with telephone queries but you can email them.

Allergy UK
3 White Oak Square
London Road
Swanley
Kent BR8 7AG
Helpline: 01322 619864 (9 a.m.–5 p.m. weekdays)
Chemical Sensitivity Helpline: 01322 619898 (9 a.m.–5 p.m. weekdays)
Website: www.allergyuk.org

Anaphylaxis Campaign
PO Box 275
Farnborough
Hants GU14 6SX
Tel: 01252 542029
Website: www.anaphylaxis.org.uk

Asthma UK
Providence House
Providence Place
London N1 0NT
Adviceline: 08457 01 02 03
Website: www.asthma.org.uk

National Eczema Society
Hill House
Highgate Hill
London N19 5NA
Helpline: 0870 241 3604 (8 a.m.–8 p.m. weekdays)
Website: www.eczema.org

Babies and toddlers

The organizations above can offer advice to pregnant women concerned about their own and their babies' possible allergies. They can also help the parents and carers of young children affected by allergic conditions. In addition, you might like to contact:

National Childbirth Trust
Alexandra House
Oldham Terrace
Acton
London W3 6NH
Enquiry line: 0870 444 8707
Breast-feeding line: 0870 444 8708
Website: www.nctpregnancyandbabycare.com
Offers help and advice for mums wishing to breast-feed or having problems breast-feeding.

National Childminding Association
8 Mason's Hill
Bromley
Kent BR2 9EY
Tel: 0800 169 4486 (10 a.m.–4 p.m. weekdays)
Website: www.ncma.org.uk
Has information to help parents and childminders care for children
with allergies.

Pre-School Learning Alliance
69 King's Cross Road
London WC1X 9LL
Tel: 020 7833 0991
Website: www.pre-school.org.uk
Has information to help parents, playgroup leaders, nursery nurses
and all those caring for pre-school children with allergies.

Sainsbury's/WellBeing Eating for Pregnancy Helpline: 0845 130
3646 (10 a.m.–4 p.m. weekdays)
Qualified dieticians offer advice on healthy eating during pregnancy,
including the latest findings.

UK Nappy Line: 01983 401959
Nappy Line Scotland: 01324 878609
Nappy Line Wales: 0845 456 2477
Website: www.nappyline.org.uk
For information about 'real nappies', including retailers and laundry
services.

Food allergies

Healthy eating for children on special diets is much easier than it
used to be. Most major food manufacturers can send you details of
which of their products are suitable for those sensitive to the most
common allergens, like nuts, dairy products and wheat. There are
also lots of specialist manufacturers producing wheat- and dairy-free
ranges of food. Health-food stores and organic grocers are good
sources of suitable products and the following organizations may
also be able to help.

Coeliac UK
PO Box 220
High Wycombe
Bucks HP11 2HY
Helpline: 0870 444 8804
Website: www.coeliac.co.uk
Offers help and information for those diagnosed with coeliac disease. This is not, strictly speaking, an allergy, but an intolerance to gluten, a protein found in wheat, barley, rye and oats.

Hyperactive Children's Support Group
71 Whyke Lane
Chichester
West Sussex PO19 7PD
Tel: 01243 551313
Website: www.hacsg.org.uk
Help for parents of children with Attention Deficit Hyperactivity Disorder and similar conditions, including advice on additive-free diets.

The Vegan Society
Donald Watson House
7 Battle Road
St Leonards-on-Sea
East Sussex TN37 7AA
Tel: 0845 458 8244
Website: www.vegansociety.com
It is, of course, perfectly possible to be allergic to vegetarian and vegan products – especially nuts. However, vegetarian and vegan cookery books are often good sources of ideas and ways of adapting foods. Vegans eat no dairy products or eggs so vegan recipes may be suitable for children who cannot tolerate these items.

The Vegetarian Society
Parkdale
Dunham Road
Altrincham
Cheshire WA14 4QG
Tel: 0161 925 2000
Website: www.vegsoc.org

Many **supermarkets** now produce their own 'Free From' ranges and can also send customers information about which of their regular products are suitable for those with allergies. Contact numbers are:

Asda: 0500 100055
Co-Op: 0800 317827
Sainsbury's: 0800 636262
Tesco: 0800 505555
Waitrose: 0800 188884

Specialist food companies producing gluten-free, egg- and dairy-free products include

Alpro – dairy-free milk, cream, yogurt and desserts: 08000 188 180 or www.alprosoya.co.uk
Baker's Delight – gluten-free bread and cakes: 0845 120 0038
D&D – dairy-free chocolate: 02476 370909
Dietary Specials – gluten- and wheat-free foods: 07041 544044 or www.nutritionpoint.co.uk
Doves Farm – gluten-free flours, cakes, biscuits: 01488 684880 or www.dovesfarm.co.uk
Energ-G – gluten-free breads, pastas, egg replacers: 020 8336 2323
Heron Foods – gluten/wheat-free: +353 (0)23 39006 or www.glutenfreedirect.com
It's Nut Free – cakes, biscuits and cereals: 01765 641890 or www.itsnutfree.com
Kinnertons – nut-free chocolate: 020 7284 9500 or www.kinnerton.com
Meridian – gluten-, wheat- and dairy-free Italian and Indian sauces: 01490 413151 or www.meridianfoods.co.uk
Plamil Foods – non-dairy mayonnaise and chocolate: 01303 850588
Pure – non-dairy spreads: 0800 028 4499 or www.purespreads.com
Tofutti – dairy-free desserts: 020 8861 4443
Trufree – gluten free bread, biscuits, pasta: 01225 711801 or www.trufree.co.uk
The Village Bakery – bread, cakes, puddings and fruit bars which can be gluten-, dairy- and wheat-free: 01768 898437 or www.village-bakery.com

Some companies offer fast home delivery of suitable foods. Try

Dietary Needs Direct: 01527 579086 or
www.dietaryneedsdirect.co.uk
Goodness Direct: 0871 871 6611 or www.GoodnessDirect.co.uk
Zedz Foods: 01691 648029 or www.zedzfoods.co.uk

Foods Matter is a monthly subscription magazine aimed at those with food allergy, intolerance and sensitivity problems. They arrange tastings of new products and keep track of research findings. Contact them at
5 Lawn Road
London NW3 2XS
Tel: 020 7722 2866
Website: www.foodsmatter.com

Hay fever

The pollen count is generally included as part of radio and TV weather forecasts. Many of the companies which produce over-the-counter hay-fever treatments have a dedicated Pollen Line which you can call for the latest information.

The **NasalAir** guard is a plastic device which fits inside the nose to filter out pollen allergens. More details from 0845 066 2244 or www.nasalairguard.co.uk.

Pet allergies

Cats Protection
National Cat Centre
Chelwood Gate
Haywards Heath
West Sussex RH17 7TT
Helpline: 08702 099 099 (9 a.m.–4.30 p.m. weekdays)
Website: www.cats.org.uk
Has a leaflet *Do You Have Asthma?* with advice on asthma and allergy management for cat-owners.

Pet wipes, which are said to reduce the allergens in pet dander, are available to help. Contact details are

Petal Cleanse: 01608 686626 or www.bio-life.co.uk
Simple Solution Allergy Relief Wipes: 01480 492141 or www.bramton.com

Environmental allergies

As with foods, many companies are now producing allergy-friendly toiletries and household cleaners. None can offer a 100 per cent guarantee that your child will not suffer an allergic reaction but if you would prefer a chemical-free home, these are the names to look out for. Products approved by Allergy UK carry a special logo. If you are planning to buy a car, the Ford Focus C-Max has been awarded their Seal of Approval!

Toiletries

A-Derma – skincare products based on oats: 0845 117 0116
Aru Herbals: 01664 420048 or www.aruskincare.com
Barefoot Botanicals: 0870 220 2273 or www.barefoot-botanicals.com
Dr Hauschka: 01386 792642 or www.drhauschka.co.uk
Essential Care: 01284 728416 or www.essential-care.co.uk
Grandma Vines: 01482 337861 or www.grandma-vines.co.uk
Green People: 08702 401444 or www.greenpeople.co.uk
Little Me: 020 8614 4700 or www.littlemebabyorganics.co.uk
The Natural Skincare Factory: 01224 633305 or www.natural-skincare-product.com
Neal's Yard Remedies: 020 7627 1949 or www.nealsyardremedies.com
Organic Blue: 020 8424 8844 or www.organicblue.com
Weleda: 0115 944 8222 or www.weleda.co.uk

The Organic Pharmacy in London's King's Road sells own-brand products and other organic skincare ranges: 020 7351 2232 or www.TheOrganicPharmacy.com

Household products

AllergyBestBuys – various products: 08707 455002 or
www.allergybestbuys.com
Dyson Cleaners – the first Allergy UK-approved washing machine,
the CRO2 2-Drums, as well as effective vacuum cleaners: 08705
275104 or www.dyson.co.uk
Ecover – range of household cleaning products with no unnecessary
chemicals: 01635 574553 or www.ecover.com
Filter Queen – surface and room air cleaners: 0800 328 3929 or
www.filterqueen.com
The Green Building Store – for green building products: 01484
854898 or www.greenbuildingstore.co.uk
The Green Shop – everything from paints to books to bodycare:
01452 770629 or www.greenshop.co.uk
Health Guard – Total Hygiene DM 1 anti-dust mite spray: 020
8343 9911 or www.HealthGuardTM.com
The Healthy House – mail-order catalogue with lots of anti-allergy
products: 01453 752216 or www.healthy-house.co.uk
Medivac Healthcare – mail-order company selling vacuum cleaners
with special filters, also anti-allergy bedlinen: 0845 130 6969 or
www.medivac.co.uk
Miele – vacuum cleaners: 01235 554455 or www.miele.co.uk
Polti UK – cleaners: 01249 815511 or www.polti-ltd.co.uk
Sebo – vacuum cleaners: 01494 465533 or www.sebo.co.uk

Air cleaners

Alpine Environments: 0113 200 8210 or
www.alpine-environments.co.uk
Bionaire: 0800 052 3615 or www.bionaire.com
Daikin Airconditioning: 01737 732345 (UK East) or 01454 281000
(UK West) or www.daikin.co.uk
Diffusion Air Treatment: 01256 814162 or www.UVGI.co.uk
essa: 08707 505 670 or www.essaeu.com
Kiltox: 0845 166 2040 or www.kiltox.co.uk
Lifebreath: 01256 814162 or www.diffusion-group.co.uk
Puravent: 01200 440975 or www.puravent.co.uk – air filters for
cars
Sharp Healthcaire: 0800 915 3015 or www.sharp.co.uk/healthcaire

Clothing and textiles, including organic cotton clothing and allergy-proof bedding

Alltec – professional anti-allergy house-cleaning service: 0800 695 0208 or www.alltec.co.uk
Astex – for bedding: 0800 838098
Cotton Comfort: 01524 730093 or www.eczemaclothing.com
Fogarty – for bedding: 01205 361122 or www.fogarty.co.uk
greenfibres: 0845 330 3440 or www.greenfibres.com
The Healthy House, see p. 93
Mandarina Textiles – for silk duvets: 0845 450 2248 or www.mandarina.co.uk
Medivac Healthcare, see p. 93
Relyon – for bedding: 01823 667501 or www.relyon.co.uk
Silent Mites – on-site mattress-cleaning service: 0845 345 2461 or www.silentmites.co.uk
Textiles from Nature: 020 7241 0990 or www.textilesfromnature.com

There is also the **Latex Allergy Support Group** on 07071 225838 (evenings) which offers support to those affected by latex allergy, including children.
Website: www.lasg.co.uk

Complementary therapies

If you are thinking of trying the complementary approach to your child's allergies, it's best to discuss it with your GP or allergy specialist first. Allergy UK, Asthma UK and the National Eczema Society can also offer advice. Make sure that any complementary therapist you consult is a member of the appropriate organization.

Acupuncture Council
63 Jeddo Road
London W12 9HQ
Tel: 020 8735 0400
Website: www.acupuncture.org.uk

British Homeopathic Association
Hahnemann House
29 Park Street West
Luton LU1 3BE
Tel: 0870 444 3950
Website: www.trusthomeopathy.org

British Wheel of Yoga
25 Jermyn Street
Sleaford
Lincs NG34 7RU
Tel: 01529 306851
Website: www.bwy.org.uk

The National Institute of Medical Herbalists
Elm House
54 Mary Arches Street
Exeter
Devon EX4 3BA
Tel: 01392 426022
Website: www.nimh.org.uk

The Society of Homeopaths
11 Brookfield
Duncan Close
Moulton Park
Northampton NN3 6WL
Tel: 0845 450 6611
Website: www.homeopathy-soh.org

Others

Changing Faces
33–37 University Street
London WC1E 6JN
Tel: 0845 4500 275
Website: www.changingfaces.org.uk
This organization supports those who are self-conscious about their appearance, including those with disfigurements and severe eczema.

Medic-Alert Foundation
1 Bridge Wharf
156 Caledonian Road
London N1 9UU
Tel: 020 7833 3034
Website: www.medicalert.org.uk
Produces bracelets and badges to alert paramedics to allergic conditions in the event of an emergency.

Quitline
Helpline: 0800 00 22 00 (9 a.m.–9 p.m. every day)
Website: www.quit.org.uk
Offers help to those trying to give up smoking.

Women's Environmental Network
PO Box 30626
London E1 1TZ
Tel: 020 7481 9004
Website: www.wen.org.uk
Campaigns on environmental issues and also has information about allergy-friendly products like toiletries and nappies.

YorkTest
YorkTest Laboratories
Murton Way
Osbaldwick
York YO19 5US
Helpline: 0800 074 6185
Website: www.yorktest.com
Can offer information about testing for food intolerance.

Index